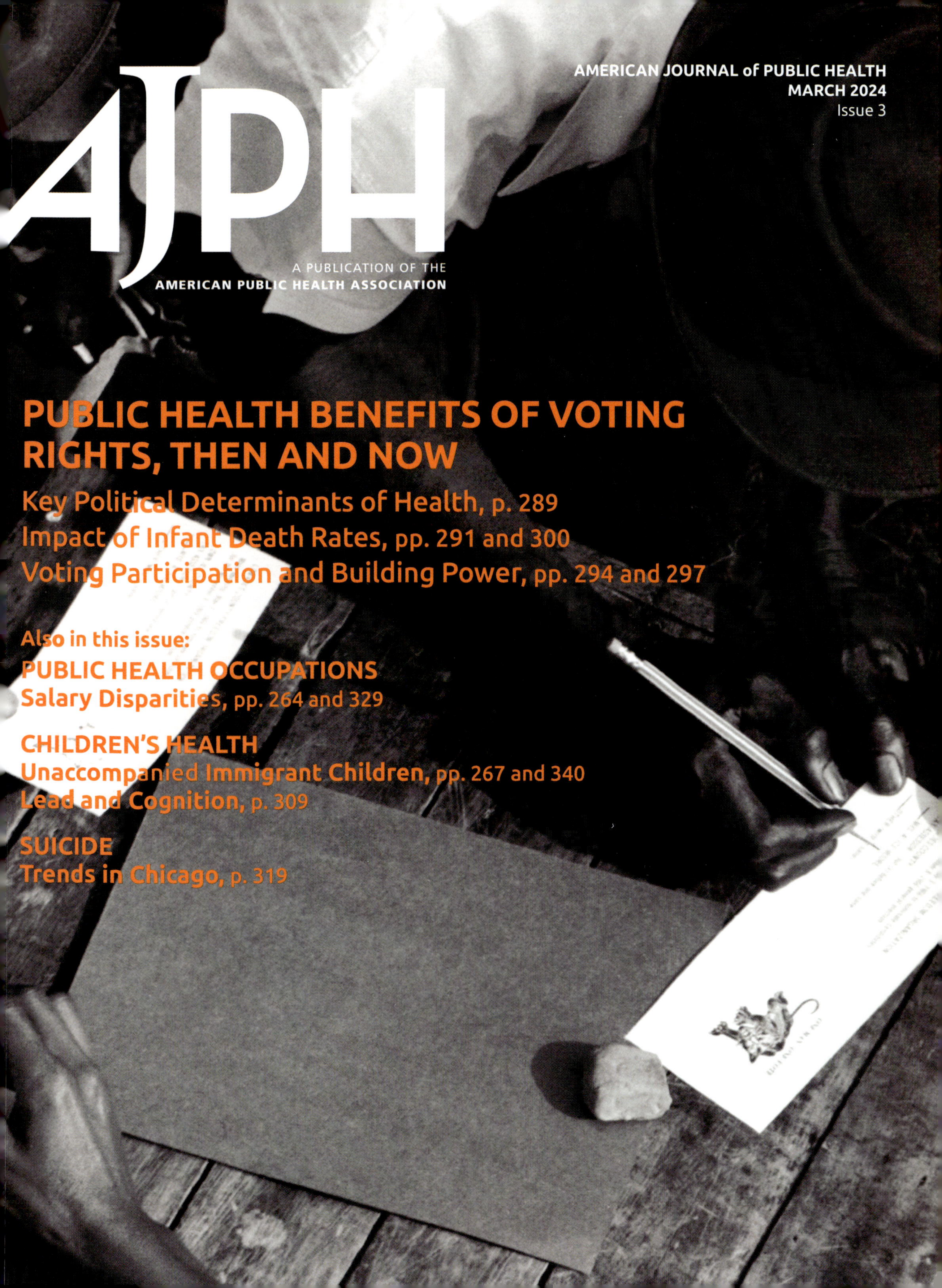

AJPH

AMERICAN JOURNAL of PUBLIC HEALTH
MARCH 2024
Issue 3

A PUBLICATION OF THE
AMERICAN PUBLIC HEALTH ASSOCIATION

PUBLIC HEALTH BENEFITS OF VOTING RIGHTS, THEN AND NOW

Key Political Determinants of Health, p. 289
Impact of Infant Death Rates, pp. 291 and 300
Voting Participation and Building Power, pp. 294 and 297

Also in this issue:

PUBLIC HEALTH OCCUPATIONS
Salary Disparities, pp. 264 and 329

CHILDREN'S HEALTH
Unaccompanied Immigrant Children, pp. 267 and 340
Lead and Cognition, p. 309

SUICIDE
Trends in Chicago, p. 319

AMERICAN PUBLIC HEALTH ASSOCIATION
For science. For action. For health.

AJPH®, published monthly, is the official Journal of the American Public Health Association®, 800 I St NW, Washington, DC 20001-3710; (202) 777- APHA; TDD (202) 777-2500. APHA is a nongovernmental professional society founded in 1872, representing all disciplines and specialties in public health.

The *American Journal of Public Health*® (*AJPH*) (print ISSN: 0090-0036; electronic ISSN: 1541- 0048), first published in 1911, is the official journal of the American Public Health Association® (APHA). The oldest and largest organization of public health professionals in the world, APHA represents approximately 30 000 members from more than 50 occupations of public health.

Submissions: Visit www.editorialmanager.com/ajph or ajph.edmgr.com for online manuscript preparation and submission guidelines. Contributions of original unpublished research, social science analyses, scholarly essays, critical commentaries, departments, and letters to the editor are welcome. Questions? Write ajph.submissions@apha.org or call APHA at (202) 777-2469.

Print plus online subscriptions: Institutional price (print copy with online access for a single institution and all authorized users, regardless of geographic location) varies by size of organization and ranges from $993–$1445 for US organizations, and $1073–$1526 for international organizations (air delivery); multiple campuses not permitted without special arrangement. Details of the tiered pricing system at https://subscriptionoffice.com/pages/apha-landing-page. To order, write apha.subscriptions@apha.org.

Online-only subscriptions: Institutional price for one institution and its authorized users (regardless of geographic location) is $878–$1307. To order, write apha.subscriptions@apha.org. For academic consortia or multisite corporate subscriptions, contact apha.subscriptions@apha.org.

Print-only subscriptions: Institutional price is US $701, $782 international.

Back print issues: A limited number of print issues are for sale. Single copies are US $49, $55 international (air delivery). Shipping included; prepay only. To order, write apha.subscriptions@apha.org.

Reprints: For prices and ordering information on 50 or more reprints, check the Reprints section at www.ajph.org. To order smaller quantities of reprints (rush delivery), use the "Purchase Article" link on the article site itself.

Electronic access: Online articles more than 10 years old are available free for personal use at www.ajph.org. Recent articles are available through pay-per-view: single PDF article for $24, single issue access for 24 hours for $33, or entire site access for 24 hours for $38.

Postal information: Periodicals postage paid at Washington, DC, and additional mailing offices. Postmaster: Send address changes to American Journal of Public Health, 800 I St NW, Washington, DC 20001-3710.

Address changes: Send to AJPH, Membership Department (members) or AJPH Subscriptions (subscribers), APHA, 800 I St NW, Washington, DC 20001-3710. Or write to membership.mail@apha. org (members) or apha.subscriptions@apha.org (subscribers).

Advertising: For pricing and other information, see www.ajph.org. Please write to ashell.alston@apha.org or call (202) 777-2470 for other advertising opportunities. Ask about special exhibit packages and sponsorships. Acceptance of advertising by the *Journal* does not imply endorsement of products.

Indexes: Publications that index or abstract articles from AJPH include the following: Ageline, Assia (Applied Social Science Index and Abstracts), Biological Abstracts, Chemical Abstracts, CINAHL, Criminal Justice Abstracts, EMBASE, EMCare, Environmental Abstracts, e-psyche, ERIC, ETOH (Alcohol and Alcohol Problems Science Database), Excerpta Medica, Food Science and Technology, General Science Index, Grateful Med, Hospital Literature Index, Human Resources Abstracts, International Pharmaceutical Abstracts (IPA), Medline, Physical Education Index, Pollution Abstracts, Psychological Abstracts, PsychINFO, Safety Science Abstracts, Sage Family Studies Abstracts, Sage Human Resources Abstracts, Science Citation Index, SCOPUS, SIIC Data Bases, Social Work Research and Abstracts, and Statistical Reference Index (SRI)/LexisNexis.

Medscape Publishers' Circle

AJPH

A PUBLICATION OF THE
AMERICAN PUBLIC HEALTH ASSOCIATION

COVER: African Americans vote for the first time in Alabama after enactment of the Voting Rights Act.

Cover concept and selection by Aleisha Kropf. Photo by Flip Schulke/ CORBIS/Corbis via Getty Images. Printed with permission.

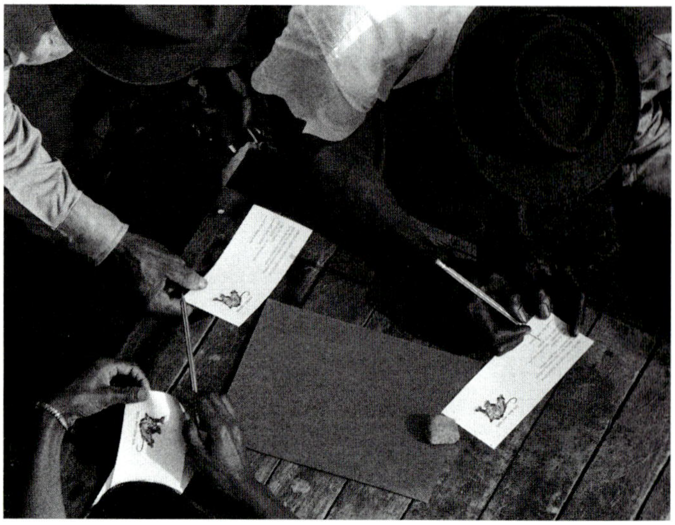

APHA
AMERICAN PUBLIC HEALTH ASSOCIATION
For science. For action. For health.

Promoting public health research, policy, practice, and education is the *AJPH* mission. As we widen our scope to embrace global issues, we also sharpen our focus to support the needs of public health practitioners. We invite contributions of original unpublished research, opinion and commentary, and letters to the editor.

The *Journal* is printed on acid-free recycled paper.

AJPH March 2024, Vol. 114, No. 3

OPEN ACCESS ONLINE ONLY PODCAST DATA SUPPLEMENT AVAILABLE

EDITOR'S CHOICE

260 The Specialty of Public Health and General Preventive Medicine to Modernize the Public Health Workforce
S. D. Turbow and R. A. Goodman

BOOKS & MEDIA

262 Oral Health of and Dental Workforce Among the Hispanic/Latino Population in the United States
L. N. Borrell and M. Makiling

OPINIONS, IDEAS, & PRACTICE

EDITORIALS

264 It Can't Just Be About the Money: How to Assure an Adequate Public Health Workforce
B. A. Resnick, P. C. Mui, and R. Maiorana

267 Protecting Immigrant Children: A Public Health of Consequence, March 2024
F. Kapadia

PERSPECTIVES

270 Black Race Matters in the Latino Population
L. Beard Morgan, E. J. Rodriquez, J. J. Juarez, and E. J. Pérez-Stable

276 An Overlooked Emergency: More Than One in Eight US Adults Have Had Their Lives Disrupted by Drug Overdose Deaths
A. Athey, B. Kilmer, and J. Cerel

280 Looking Back on COVID-19 and the Evolving Drug Overdose Crisis: Updated Trends Through 2022
J. Friedman

NOTES FROM THE FIELD

284 Training Community Leaders to Serve as Equal Partners in Research: Penn Community Scholars Program, 2015–2023
S. R. Solomon, A. Belfiglio, L. W. Tuton, and N. A. Thomas

PUBLIC HEALTH BENEFITS OF VOTING RIGHTS, THEN AND NOW

289 Voting Rights as a Key Political Determinant of Health, Then and Now
M. M. Jones

291 Safeguarding Infant Lives: The Unappreciated Effects of Voting Rights Enforcement
J. H. Rhodes

294 The Entrenched Erosion of Meaningful Participation in US Elections
J. L. Pomeranz

297 Building Power, Advancing Health Equity: Insights From Voting and Beyond
A. K. Hing

RESEARCH & ANALYSIS

PUBLIC HEALTH BENEFITS OF VOTING RIGHTS, THEN AND NOW

300 1965 US Voting Rights Act Impact on Black and Black Versus White Infant Death Rates in Jim Crow States, 1959–1980 and 2017–2021
T. Rushovich, R. C. Nethery, A. White, and N. Krieger

CLIMATE CHANGE

309 Airborne Lead Exposure and Childhood Cognition: The Environmental Influences on Child Health Outcomes (ECHO) Cohort (2003–2022)
L. M. Gatzke-Kopp, M. Willoughby, A. M. Kress, K. McArthur, C. Wychgram, D. C. Folch, S. Brunswasser, D. Dabelea, A. J. Elliott, T. Hartert, M. Karagas, C. T. McEvoy, J. A. VanDerslice, R. O. Wright, and R. J. Wright; on Behalf of Program Collaborators for Environmental Influences on Child Health Outcomes

SURVEILLANCE

319 Suicide Methods and Trends Across Race/Ethnicity, Age, and Sex Groups in Chicago, Illinois, 2015–2021
J. R. Goodwill and R. Baccile

OPEN-THEMED RESEARCH

329 Salary Disparities in Public Health Occupations: Analysis of Federal Data, 2021–2022
H. Krasna, M. Venkataraman, and I. Patino

340 Health Risks of Unaccompanied Immigrant Children in Federal Custody and in US Communities
J. Young, W. Binford, M. G. Bochenek, and J. Greenbaum

BACKMATTER

OTHER DEPARTMENTS

352 Subscription Form

The Specialty of Public Health and General Preventive Medicine to Modernize the Public Health Workforce

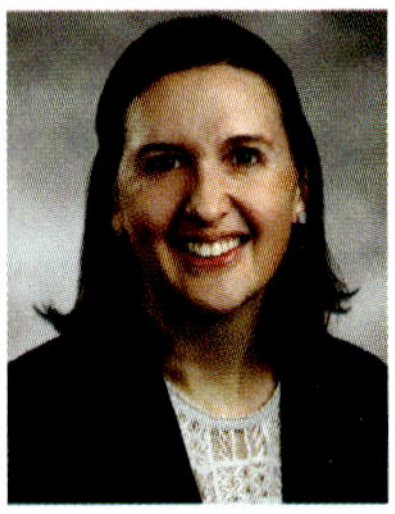
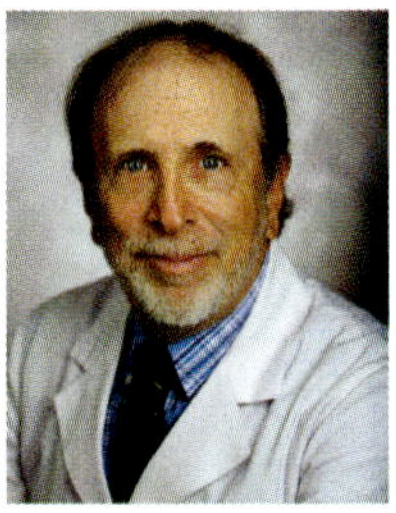

Sara D. Turbow, MD, MPH, and Richard A. Goodman, MD, JD, MPH, Emory University School of Medicine, Atlanta, GA

The public health workforce is in dire need of reinforcement. Despite the large burden of preventable chronic conditions, infectious diseases, injuries, and other major health problems, growth in the US medical workforce's capacity to prevent and control many of these problems at the population level has lagged substantially in relation to the magnitude of need. In 2007, a report issued by the Institute of Medicine (now the National Academy of Medicine) estimated that the number of physicians needed in governmental public health agencies ranged from 17 000 to 23 500, a number far beyond the 2475 physicians board certified in the medical specialty of public health and general preventive medicine (PHGPM) as of 2019. This contrasts with the explosion of graduates with bachelor's and master's degrees in public health—an estimated 1000% increase between 2001 and 2020. The medical specialty of PHGPM, therefore, can be viewed as representing a "missing link" between clinical medicine and public health. To effectively modernize and expand the public health workforce, there is a need to increase the number of physicians with training and competencies in population and public health, specifically via training in PHGPM.

Training in PHGPM is unique among both postgraduate medical training programs and public health–training programs. PHGPM residencies are available to physicians (doctor of medicine or doctor of osteopathic medicine) after they have completed a minimum of one year of a clinical residency, although many PHGPM trainees have completed a full clinical residency in other specialties (e.g., internal medicine, pediatrics, family medicine). Training consists of clinical rotations focused on preventive medicine, primary care, and conditions of public health significance. PHGPM trainees are also required to spend time in rotations in local, state, or federal public health settings to obtain experience in frontline public health practice. Additionally, trainees must complete coursework for a master of public health degree or equivalent; to our knowledge, PHGPM is customarily the only medical specialty that requires a specific degree beyond a doctor of medicine or doctor of osteopathic medicine to become board eligible. PHGPM is also the only pathway for physicians to receive formal training in public health that results in certification by a board recognized by the American Board of Medical Specialties (e.g., the American Board of Preventive Medicine), making PHGPM

Continued on page 261...

HISTORY CORNER

11 YEARS AGO

Felon Disenfranchisement in the United States

The ability to vote is one of the most fundamental rights of citizenship. It affirms one's sense of collective identity and provides an opportunity to influence public policy. Despite the seemingly intuitive nature of ensuring a political voice for those most in need of social change, approximately 5.3 million Americans, 1 in 45 adults, are ineligible to vote because of a felony conviction. . . . The rate of disenfranchisement is 7 times higher among African American men than it is among other groups. . . . Following the ratification of the 15th Amendment in 1870, which granted African American men the right to vote, the number of states with felony disenfranchisement laws increased dramatically. . . Along with literacy tests and poll taxes, disenfranchisement laws were enacted to systematically eliminate African Americans from the electorate and uphold White power structures. The laws continue to have this effect today. . . . When a group is exposed to pervasive and chronic violations of human dignity—and feelings of ignominy, disrespect, and social exclusion are prevalent—elevated rates of mortality, morbidity, and disability often follow.

From *AJPH*, April 2013, pp. 632, 633, 636

AJPH March 2024, Vol. 114, No. 3

training unique among public and population health–training programs, including the Centers for Disease Control and Prevention's Epidemic Intelligence Service Program. Because of the requirements for training in PHGPM, physicians trained in this specialty logically and arguably have unique expertise in helping to prevent and control the array of public health problems that occur in and pose threats to the US population and serve as a critical pathway to expanding and modernizing the public health workforce.

Although supporting and expanding training in PHGPM is not the sole answer to the myriad challenges facing the public health workforce, it is a critical piece of the puzzle. First, PHGPM-trained physicians are unique among both public health professionals and clinicians in their ability to work at both the patient and population levels. Because every PHGPM-trained physician also has a clinical background, they can easily pivot from thinking about an individual patient to addressing populations and can evaluate the impact of research, preventive screening, and therapies on both. This makes PHGPM graduates well suited to work as clinicians or public health officers, among other career trajectories, in a range of settings. Second, PHGPM-trained physicians are trained to use limited resources for maximum benefit; because of their ability to work upstream at the population level, physicians with PHGPM training are uniquely poised to deliver major returns on small investments.

The challenges facing those trained in the PHGPM specialty mirror those facing the entire US public health system. Like the public health system in the United States, PHGPM training programs face significant challenges, the foremost of which is limited funding. Because substantial portions of PHGPM training occur outside the health care system (e.g., local, state, and federal public health agencies, schools of public health), traditional means of funding residency training are not available for these critical (and, as prescribed by the Accreditation Council for Graduate Medical Education, mandatory) training experiences. This leaves PHGPM programs to create a patchwork of alternative funding drawn from their parent institutions, external grants, and donors. For example, of the 72 accredited PHGPM programs, as of 2021, only 17 received funding from the Health Resources and Services Administration, the specialty's largest funder. Additionally, knowledge of the specialty of PHGPM is limited. For example, some applicants to our program (the Emory University PHGPM Program) share that they have been told by other physicians that the specialty "doesn't exist." Finally, the number of physicians with board certification in PHGPM is nowhere near the size it needs to be to address the needs of the US public health system; the current gap is estimated at nearly 15 000 physicians. Although addressing the challenges discussed may increase the supply of PHGPM physicians, additional avenues to develop population and public health competencies among physicians should be pursued. These issues are significant barriers to growing the specialty of PHGPM and the workforce of PHGPM-trained physicians as well as expanding the public health education and competencies of physicians, particularly those with training in internal medicine and other primary care specialties.

We urge medical organizations and others that advocate a stronger public health workforce to include training in PHGPM in their advocacy. For clinicians who wish to obtain competencies and board certification in the primary medical specialty of public health, PHGPM training is an exceptionally relevant opportunity and should be a cornerstone of efforts to maintain the currency and effectiveness of the public health workforce.

[Note: For additional reading, see the supplemental references, available as a supplement to the online version of this article (at https://www.ajph.org).] AJPH

DOI: https://doi.org/10.2105/AJPH.2023.307568

ORCID iD:
Sara D. Turbow https://orcid.org/0000-0002-5228-9606

HISTORY CORNER

56 YEARS AGO

Compliance of Hospitals and Health Agencies With Title VI of the Civil Rights Act

[D]uring the past year (1966), a deep and significant change has taken place in the way hospital care has been offered to the millions of people in this country who are members of minority groups. In hundreds and hundreds of hospitals in all parts of the country, but most particularly in the southern and border states, Negroes are being admitted and treated as anyone else for the first time. . . . In hundreds of hospitals Negro physicians are being allowed to practice as full staff members for the first time, and what is more important, to admit and care for their own patients instead of referring them to a white doctor who had staff privileges. . . . We are still working with 100 hospitals to see if they can be brought into compliance voluntarily, and 215 hospitals have decided not to accept federal funds. . . . The road to compliance was not an easy one but change did come-significant change-and once the bandwagon started to roll it came fast and with less pain and chaos than many had predicted.

From *AJPH*, and the Nation's Health, February 1968, pp. 246–247

Oral Health of and Dental Workforce Among the Hispanic/Latino Population in the United States

Luisa N. Borrell, DDS, PhD, and Mark Makiling, DDS

ABOUT THE AUTHORS

Luisa N. Borrell and Mark Makiling are with the Graduate School of Public Health and Health Policy, The City University of New York, New York, NY.

AJPH March 2024, Vol. 114, No. 3

The white paper "Addressing the Oral Health Needs of Hispanics in the U.S.: An Exploration of Oral Health Status, Dental Needs, Utilization of Dental Services, and Workforce" represented the conclusions of a research workshop led by the Hispanic Dental Association (HDA) and the CareQuest Institute for Oral Health teams that brought together national and international senior researchers and academic advisors, HDA student and leadership teams, and the CareQuest leadership team during October 2022.[1,2] The white paper is essential for advancing oral health equity among Hispanic communities.

The Hispanic/Latino population represents the only recognized ethnic group and the largest minoritized racial/ethnic group in the United States, comprising 19% or 63.9 million of the US population. Hispanic/Latino people (hereafter, Hispanic) originated from at least 20 countries with the largest subgroups being people originating from Mexico, Puerto Rico, El Salvador, Dominican Republic, and Cuba.[3] Hispanics are younger than the US population (29.5 years vs 37.8 years). Moreover, approximately one in three Hispanics is born outside the United States, and one in five has a bachelor's degree or a higher level of educational attainment. Interestingly, almost the same proportion of Hispanics aged younger than 65 years do not have health insurance (18%).[4]

ORAL HEALTH INSIGHTS INTO THE US HISPANIC POPULATION

The white paper looks into the oral health status, utilization of dental services, and workforce representation of the Hispanic population, offering a data-driven foundation for policy reform. This work underscores the barriers Hispanic people face in accessing dental care and equips public health professionals with the knowledge to foster culturally sensitive and inclusive health services, thereby enhancing the well-being of a significant and growing segment of the American population. The onus of the dental and public health professions is to be the voice of underrepresented communities, and the findings presented in the white paper become an important tool to assert and highlight the dental needs of the Hispanic population using data-driven policies that may improve their overall quality of life.

The white paper comprises two volumes: Parts 1 and 2. Part 1 provides an executive summary of the findings and recommendations provided by experts and advisors before, during, and after the HDA Research Workshop. Specifically, Part 1 presents information on oral health outcomes and the dental workforce of the Hispanic population in the United States, an overview of the history and growth of the Hispanic population, a framework to understand oral health outcomes in this population, and the context for dental service utilization, including emergency department visits, the link between oral health and birth defects, and the dental workforce. In addition, Part 1 provides a timeline of important public policies for oral health between 1900 and 2022 and ends with recommendations for policy changes to improve and achieve equity in oral health among the Hispanic population.

Part 2 starts by providing an overview of the research questions on oral health and related to the workforce raised in the white paper, the methods used, and the national and state data sets used to address these questions. The introduction to Part 2 is followed by 13 chapters organized into four sections focusing on oral health outcomes (Chapters 1–3), dental utilization (Chapters 4–9), dental utilization and services (hospital and emergency department visits; Chapters 10 and 11), and the oral health workforce (Chapters 12 and 13). Each chapter comprises the following sections: an outline of the data set used, methods used, a summary of key findings, and a results section including a narrative of the findings, as well as tables and figures when appropriate. Parts 1 and 2 end with a list of references supporting the arguments and findings presented and discussed throughout the white paper.

The white paper underscores the oral health status, utilization of dental services, and underrepresentation in the dental workforce of the Hispanic/Latino population. In addition, the white paper calls attention to several issues related to accessing, analyzing, and interpreting data that preclude a meaningful and accurate picture of the oral health status of the Hispanic population. Specifically, the HDA research and CareQuest teams highlighted the difficulty of accessing national or state data, inconsistency in the collection of race/ethnicity and dental utilization estimates across the data systems used, and lack of information on race/ethnicity across states to document the diversity of the dental workforce. Finally, the HDA team and collaborators provided a set of public policy recommendations to improve the oral health of Hispanic people.

FROM GAPS TO GROWTH

While we agree with the information included in Parts 1 and 2 of the white paper, there are a few issues that deserve consideration for the oral health and workforce needed to treat the Hispanic population now and in the future. For instance, the Hispanic population increased from 50.5 million in 2010 to 63.9% to 2022.[5] This population growth comes with an increase in diversity associated with country of origin, immigration status, socioeconomic status and access to care, and health status, to name a few factors.[3] Together with these diversity changes, the demographics of the population are changing with the most significant changes being associated with country of origin, aging, and immigration. There has been an increase in the number of people of Venezuelan origin arriving in the United States since 2015, including people from ages across the lifespan and, thus, with the health conditions associated with aging. Similarly, Mexican Americans, the largest subgroup within the Hispanic population, are aging and have experienced a decline in immigration.[3]

These changes are directly related to the oral health needs of the Hispanic population and, foremost, the dental workforce to treat this population and their needs. These issues must be accounted for to address oral health inequities in the US population as the aggregation of the Hispanic population may ignore its diversity and, thus, hide inequities within the population. Despite these issues, which are not unique to this report or the Hispanic population, we commend the HDA leadership and the CareQuest Institute for Oral Health for a comprehensive and detailed effort to assemble the white paper reports. AJPH

CORRESPONDENCE

Correspondence should be sent to Luisa N. Borrell, DDS, PhD, Department of Epidemiology and Biostatistics, Graduate School of Public Health and Health Policy, The City University of New York, 55 W 125th St, 530, New York, NY 10027 (e-mail: luisa.borrell@sph.cuny.edu). Reprints can be ordered at https://ajph.org by clicking the "Reprints" link.

PUBLICATION INFORMATION

Full Citation: Borrell LN, Makiling M. Oral health of and dental workforce among the Hispanic/Latino population in the United States. *Am J Public Health*. 2024;114(3):262–263.

Acceptance Date: December 21, 2023.

DOI: https://doi.org/10.2105/AJPH.2024.307577

CONTRIBUTORS

L. N. Borrell was responsible for writing and reviewing the article. M. Makiling contributed to the writing of the article. The authors critically reviewed and approved the final version of the article.

ACKNOWLEDGMENTS

M. Makiling is an inaugural recipient of the Dr. Michael Apa Scholarship in Oral Population Health, supporting his work and studies at the City University of New York Graduate School of Public Health and Health Policy.

Note. The views expressed in this article are solely those of the authors and do not necessarily reflect the opinions of the funder.

CONFLICTS OF INTEREST

The authors have no conflicts of interest to disclose.

REFERENCES

1. Hispanic Dental Association and CareQuest Institute for Oral Health. Addressing the oral health needs of Hispanics in the US: an exploration of oral health status, dental needs, utilization of dental services, and workforce. Hispanic Dental Association and CareQuest Institute for Oral Health, Inc. April 2023. Available at: https://www.carequest.org/resource-library/addressing-oral-health-needs-hispanics-us. Accessed January 19, 2024.
2. Hispanic Dental Association and CareQuest Institute for Oral Health. Addressing the oral health needs of Hispanics in the US: an exploration of oral health status, dental needs, utilization of dental services, and workforce, Part 2. Hispanic Dental Association and CareQuest Institute for Oral Health, Inc. April 2023. Available at: https://www.carequest.org/resource-library/addressing-oral-health-needs-hispanics-us. Accessed January 19, 2024.
3. Moslimani M, Lopez MH, Noe-Bustamante L. 11 facts about Hispanic origin groups in the US Pew Research Center. August 16, 2023. Available at: https://www.pewresearch.org/short-reads/2023/08/16/11-facts-about-hispanic-origin-groups-in-the-us. Accessed January 19, 2024.
4. Hill L, Artiga S, Damico A. Health coverage by race and ethnicity, 2010–2022. KFF. January 11, 2024 Available at: https://www.kff.org/racial-equity-and-health-policy/issue-brief/health-coverage-by-race-and-ethnicity. Accessed January 19, 2024.
5. Funk C, Lopez MH. A brief statistical portrait of US Hispanics. Pew Research Center. June 14, 2022. Available at: https://www.pewresearch.org/science/2022/06/14/a-brief-statistical-portrait-of-u-s-hispanics. Accessed January 19, 2024.

It Can't Just Be About the Money: How to Assure an Adequate Public Health Workforce

Beth A. Resnick, DrPH, MPH, Paulani C. Mui, MPH, and Ruth Maiorana

ABOUT THE AUTHORS

Beth A. Resnick and Paulani C. Mui are with the Department of Health Policy and Management, Johns Hopkins Bloomberg School of Public Health, Baltimore, MD. Ruth Maiorana is with the Maryland Association of County Health Officers (MACHO), Baltimore.

See also Krasna et al., p. 329.

AJPH March 2024, Vol. 114, No. 3

In the article by Krasna et al. on salary disparities in public health occupations (p. 329), the authors analyzed 2022 median salary differentials of public health occupation categories in the public and private sectors using Bureau of Labor Statistics Occupational and Wage Statistics data. Ten occupation categories, primarily in management, computer, and scientific and research, had disparities of 20% to 46.9%, whereas inspection and compliance, technicians, and clinical occupations had disparities of 10% to 19%. Overall, 30 of 44 occupations examined had public sector salary disparities of at least 5%.

Salary disparities emphasize the urgency of rectifying pay inequities in public health occupations. However, many public health positions are governed by state employee pay structures that cannot be changed for only one agency. Given the challenges of increasing governmental pay just for public health, the findings underscore the need for additional approaches to public health recruitment and retention that are within the public health sector's control. Within the authors' strategy categories, additional approaches are suggested, informed by interviews with public health workers from across the country and public health workforce reports from the field.

STRATEGY #1: BENEFITS

The authors cite research showing that public health students' reasons for wanting to work for the government include job security (84.7%), competitive benefits (82.2%), identifying with organizational mission (82.2%), and training and continuing education opportunities (80.6%).[1] We recommend that agencies quantify and convey the value of governmental benefit packages (benefit reports, cost calculators, etc.); doing so would both aid recruitment of potential employees and remind current employees of the value of government employment compared with the private sector. Capturing and sharing testimonials on public sector benefits from public health workers at different career stages could be an effective recruiting tool.

Quantifying nonsalary benefits for recent graduates can help inform their decision-making as they transition from students to working professionals. For example, a recent graduate student reflected that "when applying for jobs . . . I paid less attention to things like time-off and . . . the benefits I have as a part of my position." For midcareer employees, high-quality family health care benefits and retirement plans can offer financial and well-being security.

STRATEGY #2: PUBLIC SERVICE MOTIVATION

Krasna et al. cite research indicating that public health students are willing to be paid \$17 300 to \$22 639 less annually for a more meaningful job.[2] Although meaningful work can appeal to potential applicants in recruitment postings, it should not be a sole recruitment and retention strategy. Interviewees cited a need for people-centered work cultures and provided examples such as work-from-home options, inviting office spaces, and prioritizing diversity, equity, and inclusion (DEI) initiatives.

Public health workforce development has traditionally focused on recruitment and worker training, with minimal focus on worker satisfaction. However, interviewees continually stressed the need to feel supported and valued. As an example, in data-focused positions with competitive salary disadvantages, solely training workers in data analysis is insufficient without broader engagement in the meaning and impact of their work on the communities they serve.

Although meaningful work may entice some workers to join an agency, greater focus on retention is needed for long-term workforce sustainability. Interviewees emphasized the need to feel valued and heard by agency leadership and to see a pathway for advancement. They want to work for leaders who listen with intent and authenticity and prioritize workforce development, engagement, mentorship, and advancement.

STRATEGY #3: RECRUITMENT AND ONBOARDING

The authors cite initiatives to improve the image of public health, attract job applicants, and prioritize onboarding and employee wellness.[3,4] We suggest expanding these efforts to include academic partnerships and establishment of employment navigators and mentors to help applicants with lengthy and cumbersome governmental hiring processes. For example, the Maryland Department of Health's Office of Human Resources and the Johns Hopkins Bloomberg School of Public Health's Career Services Office held joint recruitment sessions and office hours to help students transition into governmental positions successfully.

Other partnerships, some forged during the pandemic, offer recruitment potential; one example is the Medical Reserve Corps, which prepares citizen emergency responders. Outreach to this group, as well as to other entities such as civil air patrols and community fire, military, and rescue programs, could yield public health recruits with shared skills in logistics and incident command structure. Building relationships with middle and high school students and community-based organizations to offer job and internship opportunities can prepare a pipeline of public health workers. Even if these youths do not enter the public health field, their experiences likely will increase support for and understanding of public health work.

We can build on existing efforts that created descriptive job titles and posted templates for agencies to advertise for public health roles in ways that resonate with younger audiences.[3] Given limited local-level resources, marketing campaigns conducted at state or federal levels that emphasize desirable attributes of government service could help to broaden applicant pools.

At an agency level, sharing the personal stories of public health employees—from various backgrounds and serving in different roles—about the value of their work could help recruit employees and would have the dual benefit of engaging current employees in the outreach process and emphasizing the positive aspects of their jobs. Sharing these stories via social media can help reach target audiences and strengthen public health awareness and support.

More concerted efforts are needed to demonstrate a commitment to worker well-being, beginning when staff are onboarded and sustained throughout their tenure. Beyond typical employer-supported mental health and well-being resources such as Employee Assistance Programs, we heard examples of agencies formalizing leadership engagement in new employee orientation and onboarding processes to ensure that staff feel supported from day 1, incorporating mental health and well-being into staff communications to all employees, and investing in staff professional development and training opportunities. It is equally important to support staff personal health and well-being by maintaining a self-care infrastructure (e.g., organization-supported fitness programs, healthy food options). Institutionalizing worker well-being into workplace culture can help retain a healthier and committed workforce.

STRATEGY #4: STUDENT LOAN REPAYMENT

Krasna et al. note that student loan debt may influence job candidates to choose higher-paying private sector jobs. Federal data show that median postgraduate earnings for master of public health graduates were $48 866, but loan debt was $52 263.[2] Additionally, the authors emphasized racial disparities in student loan debt, which may hinder workforce diversification efforts. The Public Health Workforce Loan Repayment Program, approved in 2022 but not yet funded, would provide loan repayment for employees with public health graduate degrees working in public health laboratory sciences, informatics, or statistics positions.

Public health advocates should convey why loan repayment funding is needed and how tuition remission programs can help address workforce shortages. Adapting health care provider recruitment and training programs for underserved areas, offering apprenticeships, and developing programs to improve pipelines into governmental public health should be explored.

In conclusion, the authors' work to quantify salary disparities for comparable positions in public health versus the private sector is critical for improved understanding and evidence building to increase compensation. Given inherent governmental resource limitations, strategies such as quantifying and communicating the value of government benefits and mission-driven work to both prospective and current employees are also needed. Furthermore, creating and maintaining meaningful and fulfilling public health agency workplace cultures that are enticing and supportive to both potential and current employees are imperative to maintain a public health workforce that can adequately protect the health of the American public. AJPH

CORRESPONDENCE

Correspondence should be sent to Beth Resnick, 615 N. Wolfe St, E-2033, Baltimore, MD 21205 (e-mail: bresnick@jhu.edu). Reprints can be ordered at http://www.ajph.org by clicking the "Reprints" link.

PUBLICATION INFORMATION

Full Citation: Resnick BA, Mui PC, Maiorana R. It can't just be about the money: how to assure an adequate public health workforce. *Am J Public Health*. 2024;114(3):264–266.

Acceptance Date: December 9, 2023

DOI: https://doi.org/10.2105/AJPH.2023.307563

CONTRIBUTORS

All authors contributed to the final writing and development of recommendations. B. A. Resnick and P .C. Mui conducted the focus groups and individual interviews with state and local public health practitioners.

ACKNOWLEDGMENTS

We acknowledge the state and local health officers who provided input for this work and their continued public service and commitment to protecting and advancing the public's health.

CONFLICTS OF INTEREST

The authors have no conflicts of interest to disclose.

REFERENCES

1. Yeager VA, Beitsch LM, Johnson SM, Halverson PK. Public health graduates and employment in governmental public health: factors that facilitate and deter working in this setting. *J Public Health Manag Pract.* 2019;27(1):4–11. https://doi.org/10.1097/PHH.0000000000001052
2. Beck AJ, Leider JP, Krasna H, Resnick BA. Monetary and nonmonetary costs and benefits of a public health master's degree in the 21st century. *Am J Public Health.* 2020;110(7):978–985. https://doi.org/10.2105/AJPH.2020.305648
3. Region 2 Public Health Training Center. Recruitment toolkit. Available at: https://region2phtc.org/recruitment-toolkit. Accessed October 1, 2022.
4. Jackson Preston P. We must practice what we preach: a framework to promote well-being and sustainable performance in the public health workforce in the United States. *J Public Health Pol.* 2022;43(1):140–148. https://doi.org/10.1057/s41271-021-00335-5

Protecting Immigrant Children: A Public Health of Consequence, March 2024

Farzana Kapadia, PhD, MPH

ABOUT THE AUTHOR

Farzana Kapadia is the deputy editor of AJPH *and professor of epidemiology at the School of Global Public Health, New York University, New York.*

Beginning as a Trump administration pilot program in El Paso, Texas, in 2017, adults entering the United States without permission were detained and criminally charged, and if they were traveling with children, those children were taken away (https://bit.ly/3NykpLo). By 2018, the US Department of Justice had formalized this pilot program as a zero tolerance policy that would persecute and imprison adult immigrants. Any accompanying children of these adults would be sent to shelters, often located thousands of miles away and managed by the Office of Refugee Resettlement (ORR; https://bit.ly/3GVfv77). For the 2017 to 2018 period, the US government reported 2000 to 3000 children as being separated from their parents. However, estimates gathered by Amnesty International indicate that between 6000 and 8000 children were separated from their families during this time (https://bit.ly/4aozvgb).

Reports of lack of proper food and sanitary conditions as well as overcrowding, conditions that fueled influenza outbreaks at the time, emerged from site visits by individuals allowed to inspect facilities where migrant children were detained (https://bit.ly/4atGAfu). And in a report released to the Web site Axios, from October 2014 to July 2018, more than 4500 complaints of sexual abuse and harassment were reported to ORR (https://bit.ly/3RNbPKZ). Although several legal challenges to family separation policies aided in the reunification of children with their parents, as of February 2023, more than 1000 children—some of whom were infants at the time of separation—were still not reunited with their parents (https://bit.ly/3Rm1lvm). Since the reporting of this separation policy more than five years ago, the polarization of immigration policies in the United States has steadily worsened and the impact on the health and well-being of immigrant children and families will continue to drive health inequities in the United States.

In this Public Health of Consequence article, we consider how policies, practices, and anti-immigrant rhetoric have undermined the safety and well-being of immigrant children and their families—from the time they enter the United States through settlement into new home communities. We also provide examples of recommendations that can counter these effects and promote the health and well-being of immigrant children and their families.

PROTECTING CHILDREN IN CUSTODY

Family separation, a practice that persists today for "operational" reasons, receives little current attention but stands as one of the most inhumane policies the US government has pursued toward a vulnerable population. The trauma and pain inflicted on infants, children, and adolescents who are forcibly separated after enduring arduous journeys to enter the United States can cause lasting mental health trauma. Separation of children from their families must end.

Protection of highly vulnerable unaccompanied immigrant children requires greater urgency and care. First, to prevent trafficking of minors, the 2008 Trafficking Victims Protection Reauthorization Act requires that any unaccompanied minor younger than 18 years be held in ORR custody and not Immigration and Customs Enforcement prisons with adults (https://bit.ly/4818yxB). In addition, based on the 2008 Flores Settlement Agreement, unaccompanied minors cannot be detained indefinitely. Reflecting on the Trump administration's 2019 challenge to the Flores Settlement Agreement, Roth et al. wrote:

> We are not merely witnessing a crisis at the border, nor is the threat to immigrant children simply symptomatic of a "broken immigration system." With Flores and other protections under challenge, the rights of children are being sacrificed in the service of immigrant deterrence.[1(p86)]

Although the court responsible for overseeing the terms of the settlement

AJPH March 2024, Vol. 114, No. 3

rejected the challenge to Flores, the reality is that our policies for protecting immigrant children, both in and after release from ORR custody, are tenuous as well as inadequate. Moreover, in practice, rather than providing safety and security, current immigration policies for children can often inflict more acute harms and create lasting traumas.[1]

As noted by Young et al. in this issue (p. 340), although children in ORR custody receive medical and mental health evaluations via state-licensed and ORR-funded providers, this care can often be uneven and insufficient. In ORR custody, the acute medical needs of children, such as dehydration, exhaustion, and injuries associated with their long treks to the border, can be met. However, more serious mental health needs, including trauma, physical and sexual assault and abuse, depression, anxiety, and posttraumatic stress disorder require long-term and coordinated attention and care.

PROTECTING CHILDREN AFTER RELEASE

Once released from ORR custody, immigrant children face multiple forms of retraumatization. Because of exploitation as child laborers, inadequate or insufficient health care, food and housing insecurity, and inadequate or insufficient education, immigrant children continue to bear a disproportionate burden of harm even when they are released or reunited with family members in the United States.

Most unaccompanied children do not receive health insurance once they are released from ORR custody, and the majority do not qualify for Medicaid or the Children's Health Insurance Program. Although 34 states and the District of Columbia have adopted a provision allowing states to extend Medicaid and the Children's Health Insurance Program coverage to income-eligible children, this provision applies to only a narrow definition of asylum-seeking children. However, even in these states, barriers to enrollment driven by fear of deportation, jeopardizing citizenship applications, and lack of knowledge drive underutilization.

One specific barrier to participation in public programs that merits revisiting is that this participation may impede obtaining US citizenship. In 2022, Miller et al. published findings showing sizable decreases in Supplemental Nutrition Assistance Program, School Breakfast Program, and National School Lunch Program participation among immigrants residing even in moderately generous states after threats of changes to the public charge rule.[2] Wang et al. reported "immediate statewide delays" in Medicaid enrollment during the prenatal period among immigrant mothers as well as significant decreases in birthweight among infants of immigrant mothers.[3]

Barriers to accessing public benefit programs without the fear of reprisal in combination with the need to provide financial assistance to their families in the United States or back home drive many underage immigrant children to seek employment in the United States. Recently, the *New York Times* reported on the dangerous jobs that immigrant children engage in on a regular basis. Building roofs (https://bit.ly/3TEsAcy), working in construction and factory jobs (https://bit.ly/3RnrTlm), and even working in slaughterhouses (https://bit.ly/479zrOi) lead to the exploitation of immigrant children in the United States as a cheap labor source—underpaid, underprotected, and overworked.

STRENGTHENING IMMIGRANT CHILDREN PROTECTIONS

A recent report by the Migration Policy Institute provides a comprehensive list of recommendations that would improve the care of immigrant children, especially unaccompanied immigrant children settling in the United States.[4] These guidelines outline ways federal agencies, specifically the Department of Health and Human Services and ORR; state and local governments; and community organizations and service providers can help to serve immigrant children to ensure their safety, security, health, and well-being. Examples across these levels, and as delineated by Young and colleagues, include providing adequate and appropriate trauma-informed care while in custody and legal services, extending case management after release from ORR facilities, and working with local schools to ensure access to navigators who can provide assistance with enrolling in benefits programs.

Given the growing influx of immigrant families and immigrant children, ensuring care and protection while children are in custody as well as after they are released from custody are equally important considerations. These recommendations can be easily implemented and, more importantly, can yield better health and well-being outcomes for immigrant children, their families, and their communities. AJPH

CORRESPONDENCE

Correspondence should be sent to Farzana Kapadia, PhD, MPH, New York University, School of Global Public Health, 708 Broadway, Room 729, New York, NY 10003 (e-mail: farzana.kapadia@nyu.edu).

Reprints can be ordered at http://www.ajph.org by clicking the "Reprints" link.

PUBLICATION INFORMATION

Full Citation: Kapadia F. Protecting immigrant children: a public health of consequence, March 2024. *Am J Public Health*. 2024;114(3):267–269.

Acceptance Date: December 20, 2023.

DOI: https://doi.org/10.2105/AJPH.2023.307569

CONFLICTS OF INTEREST

The author has no conflicts of interest to disclose.

REFERENCES

1. Roth BJ, Grace BL, Seay KD. Mechanisms of deterrence: federal immigration policies and the erosion of immigrant children's rights. *Am J Public Health*. 2020;110(1):84–86. https://doi.org/10.2105/AJPH.2019.305388
2. Miller DP, John RS, Yao M, Morris M. The 2016 presidential election, the public charge rule, and food and nutrition assistance among immigrant households. *Am J Public Health*. 2022;112(12):1738–1746. https://doi.org/10.2105/AJPH.2022.307011
3. Wang SS, Glied S, Babcock C, Chaudry A. Changes in the public charge rule and health of mothers and infants enrolled in New York State's Medicaid program, 2014–2019. *Am J Public Health*. 2022;112(12):1747–1756. https://doi.org/10.2105/AJPH.2022.307066
4. Greenberg M, Grow K, Heredia S, Monin K, Workie E. *Strengthening Services for Unaccompanied Children in U.S. Communities*. Washington, DC: Migration Policy Institute; 2021.

Black Race Matters in the Latino Population

LaKendra Beard Morgan, MPH, Erik J. Rodriquez, PhD, MPH, Jordan J. Juarez, MS, and Eliseo J. Pérez-Stable, MD

ABOUT THE AUTHORS

LaKendra Beard Morgan is a medical student at Howard University College of Medicine, Washington, DC. Erik J. Rodriquez is with the Division of Intramural Research, National Heart, Lung, and Blood Institute, National Institutes of Health, Bethesda, MD. Jordan J. Juarez is a medical student at Temple University School of Medicine, Philadelphia, PA, and was completing a research year at Division of Intramural Research, National Heart, Lung, and Blood Institute. Eliseo J. Pérez-Stable is with the National Institute on Minority Health and Health Disparities, and the Division of Intramural Research, National Heart, Lung, and Blood Institute, National Institutes of Health.

The Latino population living in the United States is categorized as an ethnic group, which can be of any race as defined by the US Census. Most Latino individuals living in the United States are of mixed heritage with Spanish, other European, Indigenous, and African being the most dominant. Mixed heritage among Latino individuals varies with greater Indigenous mixture among persons of Mexican, Central American, and Andean heritage and greater African heritage among persons of Caribbean heritage.[1] The substantial presence of African heritage in Latin America reflects where a majority of enslaved people from Africa were taken. Mixed heritage, shared culture, demographic characteristics, and geography in Latin America evolved to define the identity of the Latino population as an ethnic group.

Recent estimates by the Pew Research Center suggest that 6 million US Latino adults, or about 10% of the population, identify as Afro-Latino or Black and Latino.[2] There are limited health data on Afro-Latino individuals, as health research has generally focused on a single Latino population or differences by Latin American heritage and not by race.[3] The Latino population includes a diverse group of people with varied histories and experiences, and many intersections of self-identity that have included African influence since the start of European colonization in the 16th century. In this essay, we examine the importance of focusing on the Afro-Latino population to expand scientific perspectives and to understand health disparities and clinical care among these individuals. There is a clear need for more systematic study of how Black race matters in the Latino population.

RACE AND ETHNICITY ARE SELF-REPORTED SOCIAL CONSTRUCTS

Race and ethnicity are demographic characteristics frequently used by US-based researchers to identify and describe population-level trends in health. Race is a sociopolitical construct that has been used to classify population groups based on phenotype or skin color throughout the history of the European presence in the Americas. Among persons of African heritage, racial classification led to enslavement and exploitation. As social constructs that are assessed by self-report in health research, race and ethnicity have robust associations with life expectancy, clinical events, and disease incidence in many conditions. These may reflect the contributions of lived experiences, including racism and discrimination, as well as environmental, behavioral, and biological factors. In a heterogeneous group such as the Latino population, how one believes people in the United States perceive your race ("street race") may add another component to the influence of identity on health status.[4]

AFRO-LATINO HEALTH IN THE UNITED STATES

Individuals who identify as Afro-Latino may share a racial identity with Black non-Latino persons and experience racism in everyday activities. However, most Afro-Latino persons share some amount of common ethnic, cultural, and linguistic characteristics with White and other Latino individuals within the United States. Their position at the intersection of these groups makes Afro-Latino individuals uniquely distinct. Table 1 summarizes selected published studies that describe differences and similarities within the Latino population by race. Most studies on Latino health have not addressed the intersection of racial identity, whether it be Black or Indigenous race, to evaluate differences in health outcomes within the Latino population. The paucity of data highlights the need for more research, especially as the US Census is poised to change its assessment of race and ethnicity.

Analysis of National Health Interview Survey data from 2000 to 2007 found that both race and ethnicity influence the health of Afro-Latino individuals in

AJPH March 2024, Vol. 114, No. 3

TABLE 1— Selected Studies on the Health of Afro-Latino Individuals in the United States, 2003–2020

Reference	Year	Population	Main Finding
Cuevas et al.[3]	2016	Black Latinos/as	Most studies focused on self-reported measures of health status and were limited by inconsistent use of race and skin color measures.
LaVeist-Ramos[5]	2012	Black Hispanic adults	Health behaviors were similar among Black Hispanic and White Hispanic adults, but access to care was worse.
Arias et al.[6]	2020	Latinos aged ≥ 25 y	White Latino adults experienced lower mortality than their Latino counterparts who identified as Black, American Indian and Alaska Native, some other race, and more than 1 race.
Borrell and Crawford[7]	2006	Black Latino adults	Black Latino adults were more likely to rate their health as fair/poor than White Latino adults.
Borrell[8]	2009	Black Hispanic adults	Black Hispanic individuals had a higher prevalence and odds of hypertension than with White Hispanic individuals.
Ramos et al.[9]	2003	Afro-Latino individuals in grades 7–12	Afro-Latino youths exhibited higher levels of depressive symptoms than Latino, African American, and European American youths.
Calzada et al.[10]	2019	Mexican and Dominican children aged 4–5 y	Collective Black (3 least-lightest skin tones) children had higher ratings on internalizing and externalizing behaviors compared with honorary White (6 lightest skin tones) children.
Bediako et al.[11]	2015	Black Latina mothers	Black Latina mothers were more likely than all Latina mothers to experience low birth weight, preterm birth, or small for gestational age.
Kershaw and Albrecht[12]	2014	Hispanic Black adults aged > 25 y	Higher residential segregation was associated with higher mean BMI among White Hispanic women but with lower mean BMI among Black Hispanic women.
Gravlee et al.[13]	2005	Puerto Rican adults aged 25–55 y	Social-cultural processes mediate the relationship between skin color and blood pressure.

Note. BMI = body mass index (defined as weight in kilograms divided by the square of height in meters).

that there were similarities to both Black non-Latino and White Latino individuals for health outcomes.[5] The prevalence of chronic conditions, such as diabetes and hypertension, were similar among the Latino population regardless of race. However, access to health services differed by race within the Latino population. Having a usual source of care and being seen by a clinician within the past year among Afro-Latino individuals was like what Black individuals reported. However, health behavior outcomes such as alcohol consumption, level of physical activity, and cigarette smoking varied less within the Latino population by race.[5] Other research has found that Afro-Latino individuals tend to have a shorter life expectancy,[6] worse self-rated health,[7] higher levels of self-reported hypertension,[8] and more depressive symptoms compared with their White Latino counterparts.[9,10] Afro-Latina women were also found to be at greater risk of preterm birth, delivering more newborns that are of low birth weight, and having higher body mass index (defined as weight in kilograms divided by the square of height in meters) than White Latina women.[11,12]

Comparing other demographic determinants of health among the Latino population by race identifies lower median household income, higher rates of unemployment, and higher rates of poverty among Afro-Latino individuals.[3] Multiple studies have also noted that Afro-Latino individuals' phenotypic similarities to Black individuals may place them at a higher risk of racism than White Latino individuals in the United States, which may also be exacerbated by having limited English proficiency and questioning of immigration status.[2,3,5] In the 2021 National Survey of Latinos, Afro-Latino individuals reported similar experiences with discrimination as other Latino individuals, but were more likely to report being unfairly stopped by police during the year before the survey (22% vs 8%) and being criticized for speaking Spanish in public (30% vs 20%).[2] Research has consistently demonstrated the association between experiences of discrimination and higher rates of chronic stress, poorer health, and adverse health behaviors that may increase the risk of chronic disease.[3]

Furthermore, research has suggested that the relationship between skin color and health can be attributed, at least partially, to being socially classified as "Black" by other Latinos in the United States, independent of skin pigmentation.[13] This provides evidence of anti-Blackness within the Latino population in the United States and its influence on health. However, in cross-national research in Latin America, gradients in self-reported health by skin color were not explained by self-reported or ascribed race and ethnicity, although class and color discrimination were significant.[14] Instead, the relationship between skin color and self-reported health was mostly mediated by socioeconomic status and access to health care.

US CENSUS AND THE AFRO-LATINO POPULATION

Currently, race and ethnicity are assessed separately by the US Census using a two-question format. The first question asks about "Hispanic, Latino, or Spanish origin" followed by the race question: African American or Black, American Indian and Alaska Native, Asian, Native Hawaiian and Pacific Islander, White, and multiracial.[15] However, there is increasing evidence that this two-part question is confusing to Latino individuals and that up to half do not identify with any of the racial categories.[16] In 2020, the US Census estimated that approximately 1.2 million individuals identified as ethnically Latino and racially Black, which is five times less than what was estimated by the Pew Research Center between 2019 and 2020.[2] This discordance implies a significant undercount,[17] because directly asking respondents whether they identify as Afro-Latino as a subcategory of Latino was shown to yield a higher count of individuals who identify with this group compared with using two separate questions.[2]

A study of the impact of using a one-question combined format compared with the two-question format showed that use of a combined race and ethnicity question increased reporting within the Census racial categories, decreased the proportion reporting as "some other race," decreased nonresponse, and improved accuracy and reliability.[16] Given these data, the two-question format for the collection of race and ethnicity is being reconsidered by the Office of Management and Budget (OMB) and would be replaced with a single question asking about self-identity. Administering a one-item combined question would simplify the process, facilitate estimates of mutually exclusive categories, and facilitate the possibility of new subcategories such as Afro-Latino. If this change is endorsed by OMB, it would lead to revised expectations in data collection for research. The last substantial change to racial and ethnic categories occurred in the 2000 Census.[18]

To this end, OMB released this set of recommended revisions on January 26, 2023, to revise OMB's 1997 Statistical Policy Directive No. 15: Standards for Maintaining, Collecting, and Presenting Federal Data on Race and Ethnicity.[19] These proposed changes were open to public comment, are under review by federal agencies, and, if approved, would be enacted in 2024. These proposed changes may be an important step toward increasing the accuracy and reliability of demographic data collection, especially for Afro-Latino individuals. Researchers do not need to wait until such recommendations are finalized to use the single-item question. By not waiting, researchers would have improved statistics on race and ethnicity to report within a short period of time around the enactment of the revised standards.

The Pew Research Center study indicated that when Afro-Latino individuals were asked about racial identity using the current Census-style format, 30% selected White, 25% selected Black, 23% selected "some other race," 16% selected multiple races, and 1% selected Asian.[2] Similarly, the US Census found that the overall number of Latino individuals reporting more than one race increased from 3 million in 2010 to 20.3 million in 2020, which was attributed in part to changes in how "more than one race" was determined in the 2020 Census.[20] These results highlight the importance of methods and measures that facilitate the collection of inclusive and meaningful data, which more accurately captures the intersectionality of self-identity for Afro-Latino individuals.

THE INTERSECTIONALITY OF AFRO-LATINO IDENTITY

Because of the heterogeneity of the Latino population in the Americas, ethnicity is the preferred identity for most, reflecting some amount of shared or common culture, language, and history across Latin America given a spectrum of racial mixture.[21] Intersectionality is inherent in the ethnic identity of Latin American populations given

530 years since the arrival of Europeans. First proposed by Black feminist scholar Kimberlé Williams Crenshaw, intersectionality is a term originally used to describe the simultaneous racial and gender prejudice experienced by Black women.[22] This foundational theory applies to the study of Afro-Latino individuals, acting as a vehicle for understanding the experiences of a population whose health profile is both similar and different from White Latino or non-Latino Black populations. Further critical intersections include those between race and ethnicity and socioeconomic status as well as immigration history and status. Socioeconomic status often defines power relations within society. Migration patterns, particularly those driven in large part by people seeking economic opportunities over the past 60 years, contribute new intersectional perspectives.

RACE AND IDENTITY IN LATIN AMERICA

In Latin America, primary spoken language has been the most utilized measure of ethno-racial identity, with the goal of identifying Indigenous populations.[23] Since 2000, more countries have moved toward utilizing self-identification as the primary means of assessing ethno-racial identity in national surveys.[23] Categories vary by country but may include Indigenous, White, Mestizo, Black, Mulato, and others as well as specific Indigenous groups and specific combinations of racial groups.[23] Even in Caribbean countries, where Afro-Latino individuals have a significant presence in the population, the underrepresentation of African-descendant populations in positions of power has impeded the collection of demographic data.

The historical context in Latin America is rooted in systematic racism, characterized by the enslavement of African persons and the marginalization and exploitation of Indigenous populations. Rooted in European colonialism, the societal caste system that permeates much of Latin America stratifies individuals based on skin color and geographic heritage. Spanish-born Whites sat atop of this hierarchy, followed by those born in the Americas, and with all mixtures ranked as inferior. However, some Afro-Latino individuals would pass as White in postcolonial society given their phenotypical characteristics. Such dynamics may partially explain why Afro-Latino individuals in the United States appear reluctant to identify as Black and Latino but are much more willing to identify as Afro-Latino.

The dominant paradigm in Latin America has been that socioeconomic factors are the driving force behind health inequities and accepting that the implications of race and discrimination merit similar consideration in understanding these inequities is a more recent development.[24] For example, Mexico has only recently recognized its African-descendant population in its national census, estimated to be approximately 2% of the population, despite a cultural presence since the early colonial period.[25] Ascertainment of race in Cuba and the Dominican Republic has been inconsistent and often couched as "not relevant" because of the notion that most of the population is racially mixed. Across Latin America, African-descendant individuals are generally overrepresented among the poor, underrepresented in positions of power, and face significant socioeconomic and health barriers, which have been inconsistently documented. As such, methods and measures used to quantify African-descendant populations is an issue of broader international significance, as underrepresentation of African-descendant populations in national and regional surveys limits the data that can inform the development and implementation of interventions and policies to address health inequities.

FUTURE DIRECTIONS

There is a need to differentiate racial groups within the heterogeneous Latino population in the United States, with the goal of conducting additional research. The Hispanic Community Health Study/Study of Latinos (HCHS/SOL) provides a tangible opportunity for researchers to contribute to our understanding of Afro-Latino health in the United States. HCHS/SOL, visit 1 completed from 2008–2011, is one of the most diverse studies among Latino individuals regarding Latin American heritage and continues to follow more than 9000 persons from four urban sites for visit 3.[24] An additional resource, the All of Us Research Program, has already recruited more than 58 500 Latino individuals, including many Afro-Latino individuals.

Several national-level health data sets can be used to conduct such research, although some analyses may require access to restricted data or recoding so that Black or African American race can be identified among Latino individuals. For example, recoding would identify the subset of individuals who checked Latino and Black boxes from those that indicated any other combination of multiple racial and ethnic group boxes. Other studies will need to consider adding more granular questions to their data collection methods, which should provide insights into the intersectionality of race, ethnicity, and socioeconomic status. For example, adding a subcategory of Afro-Latino for persons identifying as Latino would be a first step. Additional measures, such as perceived race, could also be included to evaluate their value to health research. Using such data to conduct analyses among Afro-Latino individuals will advance our understanding of the health of this population as well as inform proposed structural interventions. We encourage researchers and funders to identify opportunities to facilitate and support research and interventions to meet the unique needs of Afro-Latino individuals and strive for equity for this population.

As the Latino population continues to grow and the United States continues to diversify, researchers and policymakers will need to revisit the way in which race and ethnicity are conceptualized and operationalized to ensure that health interventions and policies are appropriately targeted. Failing to inquire about the multiple racial and ethnic identities of individuals in health disparities research threatens to limit the extent to which we can understand and address the needs of Afro-Latino individuals. Behavioral and system interventions benefit from tailoring to target populations, and the effects of generic policies need to be considered in this context. Improving health through evidence-based policies and practice will not occur for Afro-Latino individuals without intentional data collection. Health interventions and policies may need to be tailored, and should be consciously designed, to meet people where they are. Clinicians need to be aware of these concepts and equipped with knowledge and resources to provide effective, quality, and culturally competent care. AJPH

CORRESPONDENCE

Correspondence should be sent to Eliseo J. Pérez-Stable, MD, Office of the Director, National Institute on Minority Health and Health Disparities, National Institutes of Health, 6707 Democracy Blvd, Ste 800, Bethesda, MD 20892-5465 (e-mail: eliseo.perez-stable@nih.gov). Reprints can be ordered at https://ajph.org by clicking the "Reprints" link.

PUBLICATION INFORMATION

Full Citation: Beard Morgan L, Rodriquez EJ, Juarez JJ, Pérez-Stable EJ. Black race matters in the Latino population. *Am J Public Health*. 2024;114(3): 270–275.

Acceptance Date: September 9, 2023.

DOI: https://doi.org/10.2105/AJPH.2023.307452

CONTRIBUTORS

L. Beard Morgan wrote the first draft of this article after an extensive review of available literature. J. J. Juarez revised the first draft with additional literature reviewed. E. J. Rodriquez provided critical revisions of these drafts. E. J. Pérez-Stable made all final revisions in the text and table.

ACKNOWLEDGMENTS

The effort for this article was funded by the Division of Intramural Research, National Heart, Lung, and Blood Institute, National Institutes of Health.

CONFLICTS OF INTEREST

The authors have no conflicts of interest.

REFERENCES

1. De Oliveira TC, Secolin R, Lopes-Cendes I. A review of ancestrality and admixture in Latin America and the Caribbean focusing on native American and African descendant populations. *Front Genet.* 2023;14:1091269. https://doi.org/10.3389/fgene.2023.1091269
2. Gonzalez-Barrera A. About 6 million US adults identify as Afro-Latino. Pew Research Center. 2022. Available at: https://www.pewresearch.org/short-reads/2022/05/02/about-6-million-u-s-adults-identify-as-afro-latino. Accessed August 1, 2023.
3. Cuevas AG, Dawson BA, Williams DR. Race and skin color in Latino health: an analytic review. *Am J Public Health*. 2016;106(12):2131–2136. https://doi.org/10.2105/AJPH.2016.303452
4. López N, Vargas ED, Juarez M, Cacari-Stone L, Bettez S. What's your "street race"? Leveraging multidimensional measures of race and intersectionality for examining physical and mental health status among Latinxs. *Sociol Race Ethn (Thousand Oaks)*. 2018;4(1):49–66. https://doi.org/10.1177/2332649217708798
5. LaVeist-Ramos TA, Galarraga J, Thorpe RJ Jr, Bell CN, Austin CJ. Are Black Hispanics Black or Hispanic? Exploring disparities at the intersection of race and ethnicity. *J Epidemiol Community Health*. 2012;66(7):e21. https://doi.org/10.1136/jech.2009.103879
6. Arias E, Johnson NJ, Vera BT. Racial disparities in mortality in the adult Hispanic population. *SSM Popul Health*. 2020;11:100583. https://doi.org/10.1016/j.ssmph.2020.100583
7. Borrell LN, Crawford ND. Race, ethnicity, and self-rated health status in the Behavioral Risk Factor Surveillance System survey. *Hisp J Behav Sci.* 2006;28(3):387–403. https://doi.org/10.1177/0739986306290368
8. Borrell LN. Race, ethnicity, and self-reported hypertension: analysis of data from the National Health Interview Survey, 1997–2005. *Am J Public Health*. 2009;99(2):313–319. https://doi.org/10.2105/AJPH.2007.123364
9. Ramos B, Jaccard J, Guilamo-Ramos V. Dual ethnicity and depressive symptoms: implications of being Black and Latino in the United States. *Hisp J Behav Sci*. 2003;25(2):147–173. https://doi.org/10.1177/0739986303025002002
10. Calzada EJ, Kim Y, O'Gara JL. Skin color as a predictor of mental health in young Latinx children. *Soc Sci Med*. 2019;238:112467. https://doi.org/10.1016/j.socscimed.2019.112467
11. Bediako PT, BeLue R, Hillemeier MM. A comparison of birth outcomes among Black, Hispanic, and Black Hispanic women. *J Racial Ethn Health Disparities*. 2015;2(4):573–582. https://doi.org/10.1007/s40615-015-0110-2
12. Kershaw KN, Albrecht SS. Metropolitan-level ethnic residential segregation, racial identity, and body mass index among US Hispanic adults: a multilevel cross-sectional study. *BMC Public Health*. 2014;14(1):283. https://doi.org/10.1186/1471-2458-14-283
13. Gravlee CC, Dressler WW, Bernard HR. Skin color, social classification, and blood pressure in southeastern Puerto Rico. *Am J Public Health*. 2005;95(12):2191–2197. https://doi.org/10.2105/AJPH.2005.065615
14. Perreira KM, Telles EE. The color of health: skin color, ethnoracial classification, and discrimination in the health of Latin Americans. *Soc Sci Med*. 2014;116:241–250. https://doi.org/10.1016/j.socscimed.2014.05.054
15. Office of Management and Budget. Standards for Maintaining, Collecting, and Presenting Federal Data on Race and Ethnicity. 2016. Available at: https://www.federalregister.gov/documents/2016/09/30/2016-23672/standards-for-maintaining-collecting-and-presenting-federal-data-on-race-and-ethnicity. Accessed August 1, 2023.
16. Mathews K, Phelan J, Jones NA, et al. *2015 National Content Test Race and Ethnicity Analysis Report: A New Design for the 21st Century*. US Census Bureau, US Department of Commerce. 2017. Available at: https://www2.census.gov/programs-surveys/decennial/2020/program-management/final-analysis-reports/2015nct-race-ethnicity-analysis.pdf. Accessed August 1, 2023.
17. Khubba S, Heim K, Hong J. *National Census Coverage Estimates for People in the United States by Demographic Characteristics: 2020 Post-Enumeration Survey Estimation Report*. US Census Bureau, US Department of Commerce. 2022. Available at: https://www2.census.gov/programs-surveys/decennial/coverage-measurement/pes/national-

census-coverage-estimates-by-demographic-characteristics.pdf. Accessed August 1, 2023.

18. US Census Bureau. US decennial census measurement of race and ethnicity across the decades: 1790–2020. 2021. Available at: https://www.census.gov/library/visualizations/interactive/decennial-census-measurement-of-race-and-ethnicity-across-the-decades-1790-2020.html. Accessed August 1, 2023.
19. Orvis K. Initial proposals for revising the federal race and ethnicity standards. The White House. January 26, 2023. Available at: https://www.whitehouse.gov/omb/briefing-room/2023/01/26/initial-proposals-for-revising-the-federal-race-and-ethnicity-standards. Accessed August 1, 2023.
20. Jones N, Marks R, Ramirez R, Ríos-Vargas M. 2020 census illuminates racial and ethnic composition of the country. US Census Bureau. 2021. Available at: https://www.census.gov/library/stories/2021/08/improved-race-ethnicity-measures-reveal-united-states-population-much-more-multiracial.html. Accessed August 1, 2023.
21. González Burchard E, Borrell LN, Choudhry S, et al. Latino populations: a unique opportunity for the study of race, genetics, and social environment in epidemiological research. *Am J Public Health*. 2005;95(12):2161–2168. https://doi.org/10.2105/AJPH.2005.068668
22. Crenshaw K. Demarginalizing the intersection of race and sex: a Black feminist critique of antidiscrimination doctrine, feminist theory and antiracist politics. *Univ Chic Leg Forum*. 1989;1989(1):139–167.
23. Morrison J, Ratzlaff A, Rojas M, Jaramillo M, Lins C, Peña MO. *Counting Ethnicity and Race: Harmonizing Race and Ethnicity Data in Latin America (2000–2016)*. Gender and Diversity Division, Inter-American Development Bank. 2017. Available at: https://publications.iadb.org/publications/english/document/Counting-Ethnicity-and-Race-Harmonizing-Race-and-Ethnicity-Data-in-Latin-America-(2000-2016).pdf. Accessed August 1, 2023.
24. Pirzada A, Cai J, Heiss G, et al. Evolving science on cardiovascular disease among Hispanic/Latino adults: JACC International. *J Am Coll Cardiol*. 2023;81(15):1505–1520. https://doi.org/10.1016/j.jacc.2023.02.023
25. Puertas Cavero N. Mexico's 2020 census is the first time Afro-Mexicans have been acknowledged & counted as such. 2021. Available at: https://aldianews.com/en/culture/heritage-and-history/finally-visible. Accessed August 1, 2023.

An Overlooked Emergency: More Than One in Eight US Adults Have Had Their Lives Disrupted by Drug Overdose Deaths

Alison Athey, PhD, Beau Kilmer, PhD, and Julie Cerel, PhD

ABOUT THE AUTHORS

Alison Athey is with The RAND Corporation, Washington, DC. Beau Kilmer is with The RAND Corporation and the Pardee RAND Graduate School, Santa Monica, CA. Julie Cerel is with the College of Social Work, University of Kentucky, Lexington.

AJPH March 2024, Vol. 114, No. 3

Overdose deaths have far-reaching consequences that are not fully understood. In the United States, more than 109 000 people died from a drug overdose in 2022, placing the national total since 2000 at more than 1.1 million overdose deaths. The overdose crisis has had wide-ranging negative impacts on people who use drugs, their employers, and public health systems, but little research has explored the experiences of those left behind by fatal drug overdoses.

The prevalence of overdose loss is unclear. Previous efforts have attempted to measure the prevalence of overdose loss in the United States, but there is no standard approach for collecting this information. For example, one 2018 survey asked respondents whether they ever had a loved one or a close friend die from a prescription painkiller or heroin overdose (13% reported exposure to this type of loss).[1] More recently, a 2023 survey asked respondents whether someone in their family died from a drug overdose (9% reported exposure to this type of loss).[2] Neither survey inquired about experiences of overdose loss beyond family and close friends.

A parallel line of research with those left behind by suicide suggests that overdose loss may be more prevalent than previously understood. Each suicide death affects the lives of as many as 135 US adults.[3] There appears to be a continuum of survivorship following suicide deaths such that loss creates overlapping groups of those exposed (i.e., those who knew someone who died by suicide), those affected (i.e., those who are psychologically distressed), and those bereaved (i.e., those who are significantly impacted) by suicide.[4] It is likely that a similar continuum of survivorship exists among overdose loss survivors, but the existing research has focused primarily on those who lose family members to overdose. Given evidence of poor outcomes across the continuum of suicide loss survivors,[4] research is needed to estimate the prevalence of overdose loss exposure, to characterize the types of survivors, and to evaluate the impact of overdose loss.

MORE THAN 40% OF ADULTS LOST SOMEONE TO OVERDOSE

To address this gap in the literature, we added questions to the RAND American Life Panel, a long-standing nationally representative survey of US adults 18 years or older.[5] Our study incorporated US demographic-weighted responses from wave 14 of the survey, covering 2072 respondents in February and March 2023. In line with the literature on suicide loss, we operationalized overdose loss as having personally known at least one person who died by overdose. We asked those who self-reported overdose loss to characterize the impact of the loss on a Likert-type scale with responses ranging from "The death had little impact on my life" to "The death had a significant or devastating effect on me that I still feel." The appendix (available as a supplement to the online version of this article at http://www.ajph.org) provides additional information about the panel and our methods along with detailed results.

In our study, 42.4% of respondents reported personally knowing at least one person who died by overdose (Table 1). Thus, we estimate that approximately 125 million American adults have experienced overdose loss. The mean number of overdose losses was 2.88 ± 3.11 (median = 2) among US adults who reported ever knowing someone who died by overdose. To our knowledge, no research has evaluated the prevalence of repeated experiences of overdose loss.

TABLE 1— Lifetime Prevalence and Impact of Exposure to Overdose Deaths: United States, 2023

Question/Item	Survey Respondents, %[a]	Estimated Number of US Adults[b]
How many people over the course of your life do you personally know who have died by overdose?		
0	57.6	170 472 586
1	19.0	56 232 277
2–5	18.9	55 936 317
≥6	4.5	13 318 171
Thinking about the effect of the overdose death(s) on your life, select the most appropriate answer		
The death had little effect on my life	10.2	30 128 662
The death had somewhat of an effect on me but did not disrupt my life	18.5	54 841 268
The death disrupted my life for a short time	6.8	20 066 044
The death disrupted my life in a significant or devastating way, but I no longer feel that way	2.7	7 902 115
The death had a significant or devastating effect on me that I still feel	4.2	12 548 676

[a]Based on wave 14 of the American Life Panel.
[b]Based on 2022 census reports of the number of adults in the United States (295 959 351). See the appendix for detailed methodological information (available as a supplement to the online version of this article at http://www.ajph.org).

EPIDEMIOLOGY OF OVERDOSE LOSS

We found demographic and geographic differences between US adults who had experienced an overdose loss and those who had not experienced such a loss. Lifetime exposure to an overdose death was more common among women than men, married participants than unmarried participants, US-born participants than immigrants, and those who lived in urban settings than those in rural settings (Table A, available as a supplement to the online version of this article at http://www.ajph.org). Rates of exposure were significantly higher in the New England (Connecticut, Maine, Massachusetts, New Hampshire, Rhode Island, and Vermont) and East South Central (i.e., Alabama, Kentucky, Mississippi, and Tennessee) census divisions than in other regions (Figure A, available as a supplement to the online version of this article at http://www.ajph.org).

OVERDOSE LOSS DISRUPTED THE LIVES OF 40 MILLION ADULTS

Of those participants who reported lifetime exposure to overdose loss, approximately one in three reported that the experience disrupted their lives. We estimate that more than 40 million American adults (13% of the US adult population) have had their lives disrupted by overdose loss, with more than 12 million (4.24% of the population) reporting that the loss conferred a significant or devastating effect that they still feel.

The literature on the impact of overdose loss is extremely limited. However, there is a robust body of literature showing that traumatic bereavement more generally has negative impacts on physical health, mental health, and substance use. Existing studies focused specifically on overdose loss suggest that such exposures may increase the risk for a wide range of negative outcomes. Research conducted in Norway suggests that parents who lose children to overdose are at increased risk for external injury mortality,[6] although it is not clear whether these deaths are by unintentional overdose, suicide, or some other cause. According to cross-sectional studies, overdose loss exposures may be associated with the development of prolonged grief,[7] substance use disorders,[8] and suicidal ideation.[9] Qualitative research suggests that overdose loss populations are at increased risk for other poor outcomes including stigmatization and mental health and substance use problems.[10]

To date, no studies to our knowledge have assessed the prevalence of nonfatal and fatal overdoses among adults exposed to overdose loss. Given that people who lose family members to overdose may share genetic and environmental risk factors with overdose decedents, research evaluating overdose fatalities and other adverse outcomes among these individuals is indicated.

PEOPLE WHO USE DRUGS ARE VERY VULNERABLE TO OVERDOSE LOSS

Although not measured in this study, people who use drugs are disproportionately impacted by overdose loss. Estimates of past-year overdose loss among people who use drugs range from 57% to 72%.[11,12] People who use drugs may also be at higher risk of witnessing overdose deaths than others who experience overdose loss. Nationally representative estimates suggest that bystanders were likely present at 46% of overdose deaths in 2021.[13]

Witnessing an overdose death may be a particularly harmful component of overdose loss experiences that is common among people who use drugs. Among individuals who use drugs, those who have witnessed an overdose are twice as likely to report experiencing a nonfatal overdose as those who have not witnessed an overdose death.[14] However, it is unknown whether overdose loss increases risk for overdose mortality among people who use drugs. It is also unknown which populations of people who use drugs are at particularly high risk for adverse outcomes. For example, it is possible that overdose bereavement is especially detrimental to people who use drugs who are diagnosed with co-occurring mental health disorders such as depression and posttraumatic stress disorder.

IMPLICATIONS AND NEXT STEPS

The experiences and needs of millions of overdose loss survivors have been largely overlooked in the clinical and public health response to the overdose crisis.[15] Our findings emphasize the need for research into the prevalence and impact of overdose loss, particularly among groups and communities that have experienced disproportionate rates of loss. Future research should start with the development and psychometric evaluation of measurements that reliably capture the prevalence and impact of overdose loss. These standardized assessments could be added to existing efforts such as the National Survey on Drug Use and Health and studies funded through the National Institutes of Health HEAL Initiative. Clinical and public health research should address the role of overdose loss in contributing to the overall impact of the US overdose crisis.

Future clinical research on overdose loss can draw lessons from research on suicide loss. Suicide postvention, suicide prevention for those who are left behind, is considered an essential part of suicide prevention efforts because suicide loss survivors are seen to be at elevated risk for suicide and mental health concerns. Preliminary research suggests that there are important areas of overlap and divergence in loss experiences following unintentional overdose, suicide, and homicide.[10] Future research should focus on identifying contagion for overdose mortality, such as that seen after some suicide deaths, as well as mechanisms by which overdose loss confers risk for additional adverse outcomes among survivors, including suicide attempts and deaths. This research would not only shed light on the needs of overdose loss survivors but might also help to refine overdose risk assessments, interventions, and preventive efforts. Just as suicide postvention efforts are considered critical for suicide prevention, overdose postvention guidelines should play an important role in addressing the overdose crisis. AJPH

CORRESPONDENCE

Correspondence should be sent to Alison Athey, PhD, 1200 S Hayes St, Arlington, VA 22202 (e-mail: aathey@rand.org). Reprints can be ordered at http://www.ajph.org by clicking the "Reprints" link.

PUBLICATION INFORMATION

Full Citation: Athey A, Kilmer B, Cerel J. An overlooked emergency: more than one in eight US adults have had their lives disrupted by drug overdose deaths. *Am J Public Health*. 2024;114(3): 276–279.

Acceptance Date: November 28, 2023

DOI: https://doi.org/10.2105/AJPH.2023.307550

CONTRIBUTORS

All of the authors contributed to the development of study research questions and hypotheses and study measures. A. Athey analyzed the data. All of the authors contributed to drafting and revising the article.

ACKNOWLEDGMENTS

Funding for this research was provided by the RAND Department of Behavioral and Policy Sciences.

CONFLICTS OF INTEREST

The authors declare no conflicts of interest.

REFERENCES

1. Associated Press–NORC Center for Public Affairs Research. Americans recognize the growing problem of opioid addiction. Available at: https://apnorc.org/wp-content/uploads/2020/02/APNORC_Opioids_Report_2018.pdf. Accessed April 3, 2023.
2. Kaiser Family Foundation. KFF Health Tracking Poll. Available at: https://www.kff.org/health-costs/poll-finding/kff-health-tracking-poll-july-2023-the-publics-views-of-new-prescription-weight-loss-drugs-and-prescription-drug-costs. Accessed August 3, 2023.
3. Cerel J, Brown MM, Maple M, et al. How many people are exposed to suicide? Not six. *Suicide Life Threat Behav*. 2019;49(2):529–534. https://doi.org/10.1111/sltb.12450
4. Cerel J, McIntosh JL, Neimeyer RA, Maple M, Marshall D. The continuum of "survivorship":

definitional issues in the aftermath of suicide. *Suicide Life Threat Behav*. 2014;44(6):591–600. https://doi.org/10.1111/sltb.12093

5. Pollard MS, Baird MD. The RAND American Life Panel: technical description. Available at: https://www.rand.org/pubs/research_reports/RR1651.html. Accessed April 3, 2023.
6. Christiansen SG, Reneflot A, Stene-Larsen K, Johan Hauge L. Parental mortality following the loss of a child to a drug-related death. *Eur J Public Health*. 2020;30(6):1098–1102. https://doi.org/10.1093/eurpub/ckaa094
7. Feigelman W, Feigelman B, Range LM. Grief and healing trajectories of drug-death-bereaved parents. *Omega (Westport)*. 2020;80(4):629–647. https://doi.org/10.1177/0030222818754669
8. Afuseh E, Pike CA, Oruche UM. Individualized approach to primary prevention of substance use disorder: age-related risks. *Subst Abuse Treat Prev Policy*. 2020;15(1):58. https://doi.org/10.1186/s13011-020-00300-7
9. Titlestad KB, Dyregrov K. Does 'time heal all wounds?' The prevalence and predictors of prolonged grief among drug-death bereaved family members: a cross-sectional study. *Omega (Westport)*. 2022:00302228221098584. https://doi.org/10.1177/00302228221098584
10. Feigelman W, Jordan JR, Gorman BS. Parental grief after a child's drug death compared to other death causes: investigating a greatly neglected bereavement population. *Omega (Westport)*. 2011;63(4):291–316. https://doi.org/10.2190/OM.63.4.a
11. Bohnert ASB, Tracy M, Galea S. Circumstances and witness characteristics associated with overdose fatality. *Ann Emerg Med*. 2009;54(4):618–624. https://doi.org/10.1016/j.annemergmed.2009.05.004
12. Tracy M, Piper TM, Ompad D, et al. Circumstances of witnessed drug overdose in New York City: implications for intervention. *Drug Alcohol Depend*. 2005;79(2):181–190. https://doi.org/10.1016/j.drugalcdep.2005.01.010
13. Centers for Disease Control and Prevention. Fatal overdose data. Available at: https://www.cdc.gov/drugoverdose/fatal/dashboard/index.html. Accessed May 2, 2023.
14. Kenny KS, Kolla G, Firestone M, et al. Frequency of fatal and non-fatal overdoses and response to grief and loss among people who inject drugs: an unexplored dimension of the opioid overdose crisis. *Drug Alcohol Depend*. 2022;237:109539. https://doi.org/10.1016/j.drugalcdep.2022.109539
15. Pacula RL, Smucker S, Caulkins J, Kilmer B, Stein B, Taylor J. Family members of individuals with opioid use disorder. Available at: https://www.rand.org/pubs/research_reports/RRA604-1.html. Accessed May 2, 2023.

Looking Back on COVID-19 and the Evolving Drug Overdose Crisis: Updated Trends Through 2022

Joseph Friedman, PhD, MPH

ABOUT THE AUTHOR

Joseph Friedman is with the David Geffen School of Medicine, University of California, Los Angeles.

AJPH March 2024, Vol. 114, No. 3

Considerable advances have been made in overdose surveillance since the article "COVID-19 and the Drug Overdose Crisis: Uncovering the Deadliest Months in the United States, January–July 2020" was published online by *AJPH* in April 2021.[1]

At the pandemic's outset, there was ample concern that overdose deaths were spiking. However, this could not be confirmed using publicly available statistics, as detailed overdose death records were released through the Centers for Disease Control and Prevention (CDC) WONDER platform in yearly batches, creating a one- to two-year lag. More updated provisional trends were available, but only in rolling 12-month sums that masked month-to-month shocks.[1]

The analysis in *AJPH* cross-referenced monthly death totals through December 2019 with rolling 12-month cumulative sums ending in July 2020, to recover and make public the original monthly rates for January to July 2020.[1]

The recovered numbers revealed very sharp increases in overdose deaths in the early months of the pandemic. In May 2020, a devastating 9375 individuals died of drug overdose in the United States (Figure 1). This was a staggering sum, considering that as of 2019 the highest monthly death toll had been 6299 people.

A NEW NORMAL FOR A WORSENING CRISIS

Unfortunately, this new level of mortality did not prove to be transient. Updated numbers show that, although death rates did decrease in the latter half of 2020 to about 7500 monthly deaths, they increased again in 2021 (Figure 1). The United States seems to have settled into a "new normal," with a baseline rate of about 9000 overdose deaths per month during 2021 and 2022.

The total annual death toll also increased significantly during these years, rising 30.0% between 2019 and 2020, from 70 630 to 91 799 (Figure 1). It grew by an additional 16.2% in 2021, to 106 699. According to provisional data, overdose deaths stabilized in 2022, at 107 699.

The time pattern of shifts deserves careful consideration to understand possible etiologies. As spikes in overdose mortality during the pandemic were first detected, hypothesized causes included the following: (1) increased social isolation, with individuals more likely to use drugs alone, reducing naloxone provision[2]; (2) psychological stress leading to increased chaotic drug use[3]; (3) disruptions to treatment, leading to a return to drug use[3,4]; and (4) disruptions to the drug supply, leading to fluctuating potency and the proliferation of more dangerous drug formulations.[4,5] Each of these explanations has been at least partially supported by subsequent research.

The initial pattern of increases during February through May 2020 aligns with pandemic-related disruptions to normal societal functioning, which can be measured by proxy through cellphone-derived mobility data.[6] US population mobility decreased sharply between March and May 2020 and slowly increased over the remainder of the year, albeit never returning to 2019 levels.[6] This closely matched shifts in overdose deaths in 2020, suggesting that short-term disruptions likely played a key role. During the pandemic, an increased rate of solitary drug use was reported.[2] Disruptions to local drug supplies (e.g., through law enforcement interventions) have been shown to be associated with sharp increases in overdose deaths,[7] and such disruptions were likely widespread during the early portion of the pandemic.[4,5]

Nevertheless, as mobility returned to normal in 2021 and 2022 and these short-term factors were largely resolved, overdose deaths reached a new, elevated baseline in the United States. It is therefore likely that the underlying longitudinal factors that worsened during the pandemic years—especially the increasingly toxic and unpredictable illicit drug supply—represent key drivers of

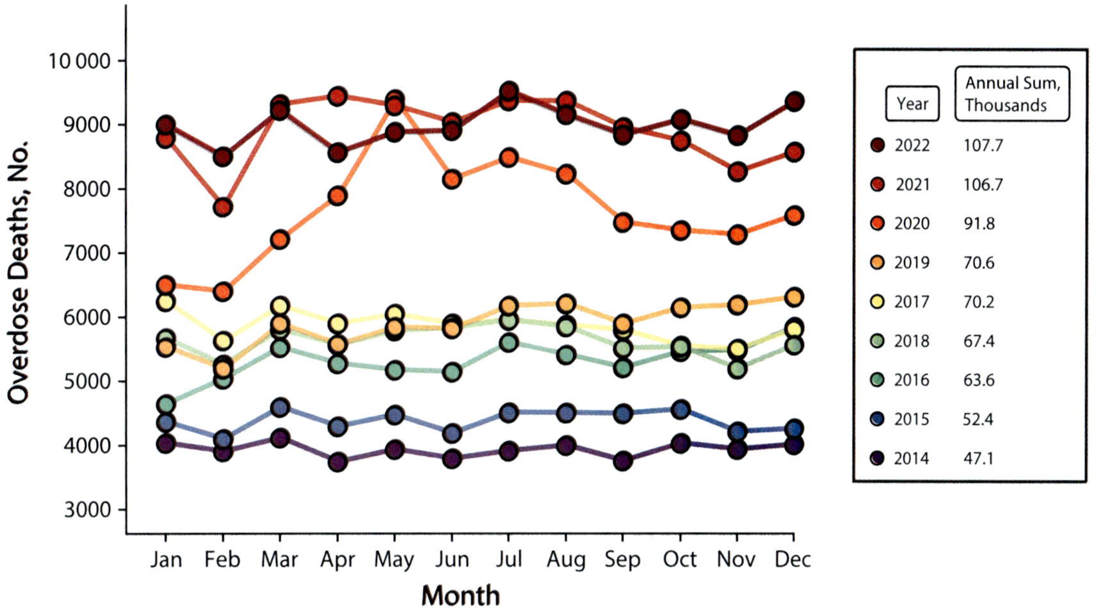

FIGURE 1— Monthly Overdose Deaths: United States, January 2014–December 2022

Note. One trend line is shown per year, indicated by color. The legend shows the color corresponding to each year, as well as the annual total number of deaths for that year. All values from the year 2022 are provisional and may be revised to a minor degree in subsequently released final values. Drug overdose deaths were defined using the *International Classification of Diseases, 10th Revision* (Geneva, Switzerland: World Health Organization; 1992) codes for underlying cause of death, including unintentional, suicide, homicide, or undetermined intent (X40–44, X60–64, X85, or Y10–14, respectively). All data can be accessed publicly at wonder.cdc.gov. This figure highlights rising counts from year to year, as well as a sharp spike in deaths during the initial months of the COVID-19 pandemic in 2020.

the escalating crisis, outweighing short-term disruptions.

The increasingly varied presentations of fentanyl analogs is a key vector of risk. Counterfeit pills have widened the market of individuals exposed to fentanyls, including adolescents and individuals seeking prescription medications. Fentanyls are increasingly mixed with other synthetic and previously uncommon substances, such as the veterinary tranquilizer xylazine, novel synthetic benzodiazepines such as etizolam, other nonfentanyl synthetic opioids such as nitazenes, stimulants such as methamphetamine, and others. Polysubstance fentanyl-stimulant use is strongly on the rise, with many individuals intentionally using fentanyl and methamphetamine concurrently, and other individuals being exposed to fentanyl unknowingly through the systematic contamination of stimulants. These shifts have led to an overall context of an extremely unreliable drug market, with fluctuations in potency and drug composition driving overdose.

In response to increased risks, many individuals have sought to protect themselves by engaging with drug-checking services to better understand the nature of the drugs they consume. Also, the widespread shift from injecting to smoking opioids is likely having a protective effect against overdose risk.

Beyond overdose, other drug-related harms have also escalated before and during the pandemic. Skin and soft tissue infections have risen sharply, related to shifting injection patterns and the composition of the drug supply, especially the proliferation of xylazine mixed with fentanyls.[8,9] The increasingly unpredictable sedating effects of polysubstance formulations can also render people who consume them more vulnerable to forms of victimization such as theft, or physical or sexual assault.[9]

Although the apparent leveling-off of overdose deaths between 2021 and 2022 is encouraging, the United States continues to suffer from an overdose death rate many times that of any other nation, and other drug-related harms remain prevalent. Restrictions on access to medications for opioid use disorder were, laudably, loosened during the pandemic, including widespread adoption of telehealth-based prescription and removal of the x-waiver requirement to prescribe buprenorphine. Nevertheless, many individuals still do not have access to treatment in a timely and low-barrier fashion, and new clinical tools are needed to respond to the unique challenges of fentanyl and polysubstance withdrawal syndromes. It is essential to continue investing in evidence-based responses, such as improved access to substance use treatment, expansion of community-based harm reduction centers, low-cost naloxone, and comprehensive housing, health care, and social support interventions.

ADVANCES IN PUBLIC ACCESS AND TRACKING OVERDOSE DEATHS

The COVID-19 pandemic also brought increased scrutiny to data transparency in health surveillance, including for overdose. In response, the CDC shortened the release delay for provisional overdose trends to six to eight months, including trends stratified by demographics and race/ethnicity—especially important given sharply rising inequalities.

Other improvements in surveillance have also been galvanized during the pandemic, including investments for state and local governments, and medical examiners and coroners, to improve the timeliness and comprehensiveness of overdose investigations.[10] However, further reducing reporting delays may be difficult. A key limitation is that the underlying investigations of overdose deaths, including toxicological analysis, have historically involved long delays in many jurisdictions. For instance, in 2015 to 2016, only 82.7% of overdose deaths were registered and available for analysis by six months after occurrence—far behind reporting for other causes of death.[11]

Nevertheless, in the context of a constantly evolving illicit drug supply and overdose crisis, more rapid surveillance would be highly valuable. Numerous approaches have been suggested, including decreasing bureaucratic delays at the local, state, and federal levels, identifying lagging jurisdictions, and funding and incentivizing timely autopsy and toxicology processing.[12] Another promising avenue can be found in provisionally coding suspected overdose deaths at the time of first contact, within days of death, supported by qualitative rapid testing that can be subsequently confirmed with quantitative toxicological testing.[12]

Additional data sources—not based on autopsy—offer opportunities for more rapid surveillance, yet are not always publicly available in a rapid and detailed fashion. For instance, the National Emergency Medical Services Information System offers a reliable and nationally representative measure of overdose trends with only a few-weeks lag[6]; however, identifiers below the level of census division are not publicly available, limiting the usefulness for state and local-level intervention. Syndromic surveillance (i.e., tracking records of nonfatal overdoses from emergency departments) also represents a powerful data stream, but improvements to public reporting are needed to guarantee timely access to detailed records.

In sum, the United States has reached a new baseline of extremely elevated drug overdose deaths in the wake of the pandemic. Great progress has been made in the speed and transparency of surveillance, yet continued efforts are required to further reduce lag times, ensure public access to novel data streams, and equip the public and policymakers with updated information to best respond to this escalating crisis. AJPH

CORRESPONDENCE

Correspondence should be sent to Joseph Friedman, David Geffen School of Medicine, University of California, Los Angeles, Los Angeles, CA 90095 (e-mail: joseph.robert.friedman@gmail.com). Reprints can be ordered at http://www.ajph.org by clicking the "Reprints" link.

PUBLICATION INFORMATION

Full Citation: Friedman J. Looking back on COVID-19 and the evolving drug overdose crisis: updated trends through 2022. *Am J Public Health*. 2024; 114(3):280–283.

Acceptance Date: December 4, 2023.

DOI: https://doi.org/10.2105/AJPH.2023.307559

ACKNOWLEDGMENTS

J. Friedman received support from the UCLA Medical Scientist Training Program (National Institute of General Medical Sciences training grant GM008042).

CONFLICTS OF INTEREST

The author has no conflicts of interest to report.

REFERENCES

1. Friedman J, Akre S. COVID-19 and the drug overdose crisis: uncovering the deadliest months in the United States, January–July 2020. *Am J Public Health*. 2021;111(7):1284–1291. https://doi.org/10.2105/AJPH.2021.306256
2. Schneider KE, Allen ST, Rouhani S, et al. Increased solitary drug use during COVID-19: an unintended consequence of social distancing. *Int J Drug Policy*. 2023;111:103923. https://doi.org/10.1016/j.drugpo.2022.103923
3. Tanz LJ, Dinwiddie AT, Snodgrass S, O'Donnell J, Mattson CL. A qualitative assessment of circumstances surrounding drug overdose deaths during early stages of the COVID-19 pandemic. *SUDORS Data Brief*. August 2022. Available at: https://www.cdc.gov/drugoverdose/databriefs/sudors-2.html. Accessed September 1, 2023.
4. Aronowitz SV, Carroll JJ, Hansen H, et al. Substance use policy and practice in the COVID-19 pandemic: learning from early pandemic responses through internationally comparative field data. *Glob Public Health*. 2022;7(12):3654–3669. https://doi.org/10.1080/17441692.2022.2129720
5. Ali F, Russell C, Nafeh F, Rehm J, LeBlanc S, Elton-Marshall T. Changes in substance supply and use characteristics among people who use drugs (PWUD) during the COVID-19 global pandemic: a national qualitative assessment in Canada. *Int J Drug Policy*. 2021;93:103237. https://doi.org/10.1016/j.drugpo.2021.103237
6. Friedman J, Beletsky L, Schriger DL. Overdose-related cardiac arrests observed by emergency medical services during the US COVID-19 epidemic. *JAMA Psychiatry*. 2021;78(5):562–564. https://doi.org/10.1001/jamapsychiatry.2020.4218
7. Ray B, Korzeniewski SJ, Mohler G, et al. Spatiotemporal analysis exploring the effect of law enforcement drug market disruptions on overdose, Indianapolis, Indiana, 2020–2021. *Am J Public Health*. 2023;113(7):750–758. https://doi.org/10.2105/AJPH.2023.307291
8. Ciccarone D, Unick GJ, Cohen JK, Mars SG, Rosenblum D. Nationwide increase in hospitalizations for heroin-related soft tissue infections: associations with structural market conditions. *Drug Alcohol Depend*. 2016;163:126–133. https://doi.org/10.1016/j.drugalcdep.2016.04.009

9. Montero F, Bourgois P, Friedman J. Potency-enhancing synthetics in the drug overdose epidemic: xylazine ("tranq"), fentanyl, methamphetamine, and the displacement of heroin in Philadelphia and Tijuana. *J Illicit Econ Dev.* 2022;4(2):204–222. https://doi.org/10.31389/jied.122
10. Centers for Disease Control and Prevention, Injury Center. Drug overdose. Enhanced state opioid overdose surveillance. October 15, 2020. Available at: https://www.cdc.gov/drugoverdose/foa/state-opioid-mm.html. Accessed February 13, 2021.
11. Spencer MR. Timeliness of death certificate data for mortality surveillance and provisional estimates. *CDC Vital Statistics Rapid Release*. Published online 2016:8. Available at: https://www.cdc.gov/nchs/data/vsrr/VSRR009-508.pdf. Accessed September 1, 2023.
12. Fliss MD, Cox ME, Dorris SW, Austin AE. Timely overdose death reporting is challenging but we must do better. *Am J Public Health.* 2021;111(7):1194–1196. https://doi.org/10.2105/AJPH.2021.306332

Training Community Leaders to Serve as Equal Partners in Research: Penn Community Scholars Program, 2015–2023

Sara R. Solomon, MPH, RD, Andrew Belfiglio, MPH, Lucy Wolf Tuton, PhD, and Nicole A. Thomas, MBA, CDP

An implementation and effectiveness evaluation of the Community Scholars Program was conducted at the University of Pennsylvania to enhance community capacity to collaborate with academics in mutually beneficial, equitable, and transformative research. Mixed methods were employed using administrative data, surveys, and key informant interviews. Participants expressed high satisfaction, valued interactive learning, and identified areas for improvement. The program increased knowledge and self-confidence in research-related skills and trust in the research process. The program serves as an institutional model to create long-term, mutually beneficial community–academic partnerships. (*Am J Public Health*. 2024;114(3):284–288. https://doi.org/10.2105/AJPH.2023.307549)

AJPH March 2024, Vol. 114, No. 3

The Penn Community Scholars Program is an intervention aimed at enhancing the research capabilities of community-based organizations. The program equips community partners with skills to become equal contributors, leveraging their unique insights and fostering equitable collaboration by understanding and engaging effectively in the research process.

INTERVENTION AND IMPLEMENTATION

The program consists of 12 two-hour evening training sessions over two academic semesters, covering topics related to community–academic partnerships and steps in the research process focusing on community-based participatory research. The lead facilitator, a community resident with a long history of family activism and knowledge of community needs, collaborated with a public health practitioner and faculty member to develop training. These sessions were iterated from 2015 to 2018 with community input. Each session includes skill-building activities, group interaction, and expert facilitation. The program engages content experts, provides networking opportunities among peers, and conducts individual coaching sessions. The program culminates in participants presenting their project idea and research questions in an oral pitch at a public symposium. The pitch serves as a blueprint for future proposals; participants have been successful at receiving funding ranging from institutional $10 000 pilot grants to larger foundation and federal grants (e.g., Patient-Centered Outcomes Research Institute).

PLACE, TIME, AND PERSONS

The Penn Community Scholars Program was implemented in 2015 out of an academic institution in Philadelphia, Pennsylvania and has provided training to 76 individuals representing 65 community-oriented organizations, all of which serve local communities in Philadelphia. Overall, the majority of participants (73%) are female and approximately half of the participants are Black or African American (48%), followed by White (42%). Approximately 48% of organizations have fewer than 20 employees, 29% are medium organizations with 20 to 50 employees and volunteers, and 23% are large organizations with over 50 members.

Most organizations focus on serving minority populations living at or below the poverty level, representing different racial and ethnic groups. By design, organizations center their efforts on a broad range of topics largely around the social determinants of health, such as education, housing, employment, food security, unintentional injuries, and violence. Program sessions are in a hybrid format, occurring both virtually and in person at the institution.

PURPOSE

For community–academic partnerships to be effective, community organizations need the capacity to actively participate in and colead research collaborations.[1–3] Moreover, the establishment of trust is imperative for fostering meaningful partnerships, especially in light of the historical mistrust that has persisted among communities regarding participation in research.[4,5] To address these challenges, the program was designed to bridge knowledge and skills gaps, foster trust, and enhance the community's ability to colead the research process. Central to the program's purpose was recognition of the value that community members bring, including unique insights into local needs, concerns, and cultural nuances.[5,6] Furthermore, the program recognized that investing in training and skill development for community members could lead to effective and sustainable community–academic collaborations, ultimately advancing health equity and improving community health.

EVALUATION

The evaluation focused on both the implementation and effectiveness of the program. The evaluation does not encompass the initial two years (designated as pilot years) or the year 2020, which was disrupted by the COVID-19 pandemic. Outcomes at the individual level included participation, satisfaction, knowledge, attitudes, and self-confidence (Figure 1). At the organizational level, the evaluation examined changes in research infrastructure and the growth of academic partnerships. Surveys were conducted after each session, as well as a pre- and postprogram survey and key-informant interviews. Surveys measured self-reported increases in knowledge and self-confidence across various aspects of community-based participatory research and program components, such as taking the lead in the research process, partnering with academics, developing goals, and creating an oral funding pitch. Surveys also measured attitudes (e.g., trust), beliefs (e.g., importance), desires, and behavioral intentions to conduct research. Participants' self-reported variables were based on a five-point Likert scale, with 5 being the most favorable.

Overall, participants reported high satisfaction, with an average satisfaction score of 4.7 out of 5. Participant feedback highlighted several positive aspects of the program, including learning, interactive sessions, networking opportunities, feedback from

AJPH March 2024, Vol. 114, No. 3

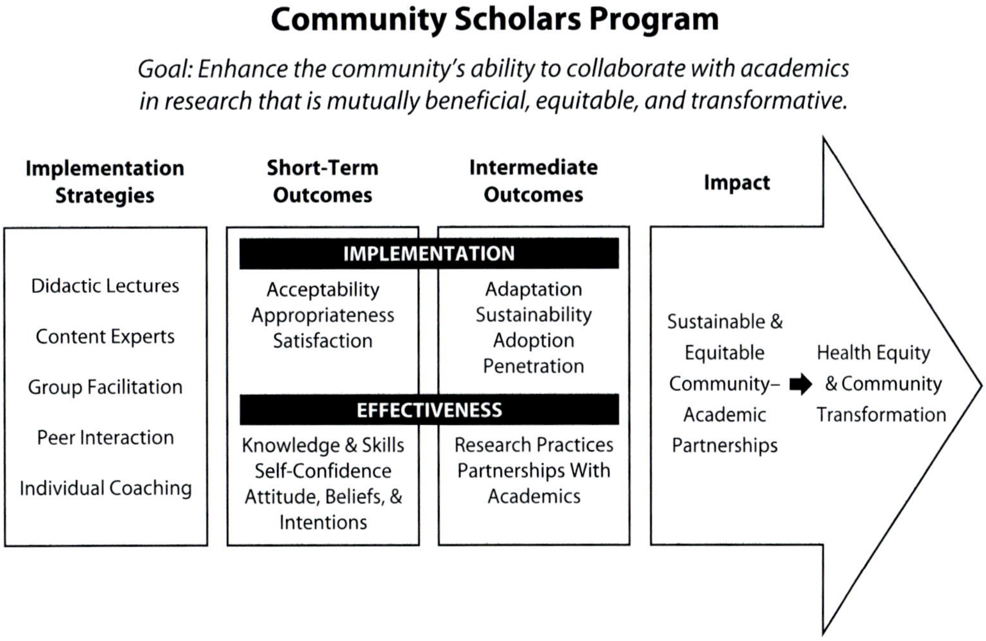

FIGURE 1— Conceptual Framework for the Penn Community Scholars Program: Philadelphia, PA

facilitators, and the expertise shared by speakers. They found the information provided to be practical and applicable to their work. Areas for improvement included a need for more time, structured feedback systems, clearer instructions and objectives, increased collaboration and networking opportunities, more advanced content, and sustained interactive elements throughout the course.

There were statistically significant pre- to postprogram increases across all variables related to knowledge, self-confidence, attitudes, and beliefs (Table 1). The largest increases in knowledge were seen in developing specific aims (mean difference = 2.4; 95% confidence interval [CI] = 1.6, 3.2) and pitching a proposal (mean difference = 2.2; 95% CI = 1.6, 2.8).

There were also positive changes in self-confidence, with the largest increases in developing specific aims (mean difference = 2.1; 95% CI = 1.4, 2.5), navigating the institutional review board (mean difference = 1.6; 95% CI = 1.0, 2.2), and partnering with an academic (mean difference = 1.4; 95% CI = 1.0, 1.9). Increases were also observed in participants' attitude toward

TABLE 1— Short-Term Effectiveness Outcomes in Self-Reported Knowledge, Confidence, Attitudes, and Beliefs Before and After the Penn Community Scholars Program: Philadelphia, PA, 2018–2023

	Mean Response		Mean Difference From Pre- to Postsurvey (95% CI)[a]
	Presurvey	Postsurvey	
Self-perceived knowledge			
Developing a research question	2.8	4.4	1.6 (1.1, 2.0)
Navigating the IRB	2.7	3.8	1.1 (0.4, 1.7)
Data collection approaches	3.1	4.1	1.0 (0.3, 1.5)
Partnering with an academic	2.9	4.1	1.2 (0.7, 1.7)
Communicating findings	3.1	4.0	0.9 (0.5, 1.4)
Identifying funding mechanisms	2.9	3.8	0.9 (0.3, 1.5)
Developing a logic model	2.5	4.5	2.0 (1.2, 2.7)
Developing a MOU	2.1	4.1	2.0 (1.2, 2.9)
Developing specific aims	1.5	3.9	2.4 (1.6, 3.2)
Pitching a proposal	2.6	4.8	2.2 (1.6, 2.8)
Self-perceived confidence			
Developing a research question	3.2	4.3	1.1 (0.7, 1.6)
Navigating the IRB	2.4	4.0	1.6 (1.0, 2.2)
Data collection approaches	3.0	4.2	1.2 (0.7, 1.7)
Partnering with an academic	3.0	4.4	1.4 (1.0, 1.9)
Communicating findings	3.6	4.6	1.0 (1.0, 2.2)
Identifying funding mechanisms	2.8	4.1	1.3 (0.6, 1.9)
Developing a logic model	2.9	4.2	1.3 (0.8, 1.9)
Developing a MOU	3.0	3.5	0.5 (−0.1, 1.1)
Developing specific aims	2.0	4.1	2.1 (1.4, 2.5)
Pitching a proposal	2.9	4.2	1.3 (0.9, 1.7)
Attitudes and beliefs			
Importance of research to fulfill organizational needs	3.7	4.7	1.0 (0.5, 1.4)
Desire to partner with an academic in research	3.8	4.4	0.6 (0.2, 1.0)
Trust in academic partnerships to support organizational mission	3.3	4.3	1.0 (0.1, 1.9)
Trust in research process to support organizational mission	3.5	4.1	0.6 (0.1 1.1)

Note. CI = confidence interval; IRB = institutional review board; MOU = memorandum of understanding. Survey items were based on 5-point Likert scales for each category from 1 = not at all (knowledgeable, confident, important, desirable) to 5 = extremely (knowledgeable, confident, important, desirable). The sample size was n = 40.
[a]All *P* values are < .001 based on paired 2-sample for means t-test.

the importance of research to fulfill organizational needs (mean difference = 1.0; 95% CI = 0.5, 1.4) and trust in academic partnerships to support their organizational mission (mean difference = 1.0; 95% CI = 0.1, 1.9).

The majority (80%) of organizations (n = 65) expressed an interest in partnering in research after completing the program. Based on available data, 18 of all participating organizations (28%) have formed community–academic partnerships since completing the program. These partnerships encompass a range of activities, including recruiting study participants, serving as data collection sites, assisting with outreach and dissemination of results, providing input on outreach procedures, and serving as coinvestigators on grants.

SUSTAINABILITY

The program's sustainability relies on continuous institutional support and has shown consistent demand from community organizations. After being founded with funding from the Robert Wood Johnson foundation, it is currently offered annually with funding from the University of Pennsylvania Office of the Vice Provost of Research (OVPR) through June 2024. Advanced programming is currently being developed to enhance sustainability by streamlining the partnership process, making it easier and more efficient for community organizations to collaborate with academics after completing the program. This initiative, named REACH (Research and Equity in Academic-Community Partnerships for Health), is also funded by the OVPR and was launched in October 2023.[7] With continued institutional support and improved infrastructure, the program demonstrates promising signs of long-term success in fostering collaborations and addressing health disparities. However, to fully assess its lasting impact, additional evaluation will be required to measure the program's effects over an extended period.

PUBLIC HEALTH SIGNIFICANCE

The Penn Community Scholars Program plays a crucial role in fostering collaboration and strengthening the capacity of community organizations to be equal partners in research. By building the capacity of these organizations and recognizing their unique contributions to research, the program enables more inclusive and impactful outcomes. This is particularly important because an increasing number of funders now require such partnerships, emphasizing the importance of equitably involving communities in the research process. To increase the program's impact on public health and promote health equity and community transformation, it is essential to advance institutional practices and academic training in the field of equitable community–academic partnerships. This will contribute to strengthening the foundation for collaborative research efforts.

Working toward a robust evaluation and continuous improvement, the Penn Community Scholars Program serves as an evidence-based model for other academic institutions interested in supporting impactful community–academic partnerships. AJPH

ABOUT THE AUTHORS

Sara R. Solomon, Andrew Belfiglio, Lucy Wolf Tuton, and Nicole A. Thomas are with the Perelman School of Medicine, University of Pennsylvania, Philadelphia.

CORRESPONDENCE

Correspondence should be sent to Sara Solomon, 929 Blockley Hall, 423 Guardian Dr, Philadelphia, PA 19119 (e-mail: sarasol@upenn.edu). Reprints can be ordered at http://www.ajph.org by clicking the "Reprints" link.

PUBLICATION INFORMATION

Full Citation: Solomon SR, Belfiglio A, Tuton LW, Thomas NA. Training community leaders to serve as equal partners in research: Penn Community Scholars Program, 2015–2023. *Am J Public Health*. 2024;114(3):284–288.

Acceptance Date: November 25, 2023.

DOI: https://doi.org/10.2105/AJPH.2023.307549

CONTRIBUTORS

S. R. Solomon drafted the manuscript, performed analysis, and played a pivotal role in conceptualizing and organizing the article's content. S. R. Solomon and N. A. Thomas co-direct the training program. N. A. Thomas contributed to the article's conceptualization, offering valuable insights and ideas that shaped the direction of the study. She also played a significant role in reviewing and refining the article, ensuring its accuracy, clarity, and relevance. Additionally, her contributions enriched the analysis and discussion of the training program's implications. A. Belfiglio made substantial contributions through his detailed review and editing of the article. His efforts ensured the article's coherence, consistency, and adherence to academic standards. He also assisted in creating clear and effective data visualizations, enhancing the paper's presentation. L. Tuton played a supervisory role throughout the article's development, providing guidance and oversight to the team. Her expertise ensured the article's alignment with scholarly standards and its contribution to the field. She also provided edits, refining the paper's language, structure, and overall quality.

ACKNOWLEDGMENTS

The Penn Community Scholars is supported by the Office of the Vice Provost for Research. Some authors were supported by the Centers for Disease Control and Prevention's National Center for Injury Prevention and Control's Injury Center Research Center (grant 5R49 CE003083).

We acknowledge the Penn Community Scholars Alumni, who are a constant source of inspiration and innovation to the pursuit of health and health equity. We also acknowledge the research assistants that have contributed to the project management and administration for the Penn Community Scholars Program, and are grateful to the guest lecturers that contribute to the design and delivery of the curriculum.

CONFLICTS OF INTEREST

The authors have no conflicts of interest to disclose.

HUMAN PARTICIPANT PROTECTION

All data in this analysis were deidentified and therefore exempt from institutional review board review.

REFERENCES

1. Coombe CM, Schulz AJ, Guluma L, et al. Enhancing capacity of community–academic partnerships to achieve health equity: results from the CBPR Partnership Academy. *Health Promot Pract.* 2020; 21(4):552–563. https://doi.org/10.1177/1524839918818830
2. Oetzel JG, Boursaw B, Magarati M, et al. Exploring theoretical mechanisms of community-engaged research: a multilevel cross-sectional national study of structural and relational practices in community–academic partnerships. *Int J Equity Health.* 2022;21(1):59. https://doi.org/10.1186/s12939-022-01663-y
3. Sánchez V, Sanchez-Youngman S, Dickson E, et al. CBPR implementation framework for community–academic partnerships. *Am J Community Psychol.* 2021;67(3–4):284–296. https://doi.org/10.1002/ajcp.12506
4. Ortiz K, Nash J, Shea L, et al. Partnerships, processes, and outcomes: a health equity–focused scoping meta-review of community-engaged scholarship. *Annu Rev Public Health.* 2020;41(1):177–199. https://doi.org/10.1146/annurev-publhealth-040119-094220
5. Brush BL, Mentz G, Jensen M, et al. Success in long-standing community-based participatory research (CBPR) partnerships: a scoping literature review. *Health Educ Behav.* 2020;47(4):556–568. https://doi.org/10.1177/1090198119882989
6. Belone L, Lucero JE, Duran B, et al. Community-based participatory research conceptual model: community partner consultation and face validity. *Qual Health Res.* 2016;26(1):117–135. https://doi.org/10.1177/1049732314557084
7. REACH home page. Available at: https://reachpenn.com. Accessed January 14, 2024.

Voting Rights as a Key Political Determinant of Health, Then and Now

Marian Moser Jones, PhD, MPH

ABOUT THE AUTHOR

Marian Moser Jones is with the Department of Health Services Management & Policy and History, The Ohio State University, Columbus. She is also Historical Editor for AJPH.

See also Public Health Benefits of Voting Rights, Then and Now, pp. 291–308.

In fall 1959, Black tenant farmers in Fayette County, Tennessee, were evicted from their homes and the land they worked because they had gone to the county courthouse to register to vote. Refusing to be chased away, the group erected a "freedom tent city" on donated land while seeking redress from the federal government. Local White people retaliated by refusing to sell them food, medicine, or basic supplies and trying to kill one of their leaders, John McFerrin, by running him over with a truck. They persisted in their efforts, living in floorless tents, "surrounded by inches of mud and mire" according to civil rights activist Ella Baker, who visited them in 1961.[1] The NAACP (National Association for the Advancement of Colored People), the Congress on Racial Equality, the Student Nonviolent Coordinating Committee, and labor unions, meanwhile, raised funds to provide for the tent city residents' needs. For young Student Nonviolent Coordinating Committee organizers such as John Lewis, who became involved in this support campaign, the Fayette tent city brought home the reality that Southern Black Americans' fight for voting rights was above all a struggle for their collective survival.[1] In March 1965, Lewis and other Student Nonviolent Coordinating Committee leaders went on to organize the voting rights march from Selma to Montgomery, Alabama, that culminated in the nationally televised "Bloody Sunday" attack by club-wielding state troopers at the Edmund Pettus Bridge and spurred passage of the federal Voting Rights Act (VRA).[2]

In the decades since the VRA's passage, the understanding of the civil rights movement as fundamentally a fight for better and healthier Black lives has receded from popular memory in favor of revisionist narratives that cast it as a campaign for equal rights under the law.[3] The article by Rushovich et al. in the current issue of *AJPH* (p. 300) brings forth new evidence to highlight the historical importance of civil rights legislation as an effective mechanism for Black Americans to secure access to the basic conditions necessary for supporting life and health. In their main analysis, the authors compare infant death rates in two groups of US counties—those where the VRA's provisions were implemented and those where they were not—for the period immediately before the passage of the VRA (from 1959 to 1965) and the period immediately after its implementation (1966–1970). Controlling for population size and other county characteristics, including health systems, they found that the Black (but not White) infant death rates decreased 17.3% more in the VRA-exposed counties (those where the federal government intervened to remove racist voter suppression policies) than in non–VRA-exposed counties during the period of analysis.

Because of the recent weakening of the VRA, these findings hold renewed relevance. The editorials in this issue by Pomeranz (p. 294), Rhodes (p. 291), and Hing (p. 297) discuss the implications of the article by Rushovich et al. in light of the US Supreme Court's 2013 decision in *Shelby County v Holder*, which invalidated the VRA's preclearance provision—a requirement that the federal government approve all proposed changes to voting policies in states and counties where systematic voter disenfranchisement has occurred. As Hing notes, the end of preclearance opened the way for a slew of new restrictions on voting: she cites the fact that 29 states, including 11 where any changes to voting laws would have required federal preclearance, have in the years since *Shelby v Holder* passed 94 restrictive voting laws. Among these, felony disenfranchisement laws and voter identification laws "disproportionately disenfranchise voters racialized as Black." Pomeranz additionally calls attention to state practices that have made voting more difficult, such as Georgia's decision to close 10% of its voting locations in the decade since *Shelby v Holder*, despite experiencing increased voter registration, and the resulting hours-long wait times in predominantly non-White communities.

Although the history of the VRA is firmly anchored in the Black civil rights movement, Pomeranz also emphasizes the effect that retrenchment of the VRA's provisions has had on Indigenous communities. North Dakota, for example, enacted voter ID laws in 2018 that expressly prohibit the use of PO boxes as addresses in voter registration, although (or perhaps because) many people living on reservations use PO boxes as mailing addresses. This matters to public health, Pomeranz argues, because "voting is pivotal for community self-determination and to elect policymakers who will address structural inequalities and protect low-resourced and minoritized communities" (p. 294). Hing is more blunt: "Restrictions to voting that target racialized voters are fundamentally about power: who can wield power and what that power can be used to achieve" (p. 298). Enfranchisement of Black persons and members of other minoritized communities grants these communities access to formal channels of power. Although access to voting may not be a sufficient means for minoritized communities to achieve health equity (and Hing argues that it is not), the articles in this issue show that it can be useful.

On a broader theoretical level, the Rushovich et al. article and accompanying editorials highlight the importance of emphasizing the political determinants of health in US public health research, advocacy, and practice. Although the public health sector worldwide has widely embraced and investigated the social determinants of health—defined by the US Centers for Disease Control and Prevention as "the conditions in which people are born, grow, work, live, and age" and the "forces and systems shaping the conditions of daily life" (https://www.cdc.gov/about/sdoh/index.html)—some interpretations of the social determinants of health have vaguely characterized conditions and systems as inevitable and static contexts while obscuring the role of specific historical actors and institutions in deliberately producing and perpetuating grossly unequal conditions and systems to further their own narrow interests.[4] As Navarro has argued, applications of the social determinants of health have avoided "the category of power (class power, as well as gender, race, and national power) and how power is produced and reproduced in political institutions" and speak "of policies without touching on politics."[5] The article by Rushovich et al. and the accompanying editorials forcefully demonstrate that these historical and contemporary power relationships must be foregrounded explicitly in any application of the social determinants of health if the model is to remain meaningful. In the US context especially, political power, through access to voting and other means, remains a vital social determinant of health.

Finally, the editorials in this issue argue that campaigns for voting rights rightly belong in the realm of public health advocacy. As Rhodes and Pomeranz discuss, efforts are ongoing in many jurisdictions to gerrymander political districts and impose an array of restrictions on voters, and the overall US political system remains fragile in the wake of the 2020 presidential election. With the reinstatement of federal preclearance unlikely in the near future, some states have responded by passing state VRAs, Rhodes notes. He argues that public health advocates should join lobbying efforts for the passage of additional state VRAs to secure voting rights for minoritized groups. Although public health advocates may be tempted to "stay in our lane" and focus solely on more direct measures to improve population health outcomes, the articles by Rushovich et al., Hing, Rhodes, and Pomeranz powerfully advance the case that securing democracy is foundational to safeguarding the public's health. AJPH

CORRESPONDENCE

Correspondence should be sent to Marian Moser Jones The Ohio State University College of Public Health, Health Services Management and Policy, 359F Cunz Hall, 1841 Neil Avenue, Columbus, Ohio 43210 (e-mail: Jones.7849@osu.edu). Reprints can be ordered at http://www.ajph.org by clicking the "Reprints" link.

PUBLICATION INFORMATION

Full Citation: Jones MM. Voting rights as a key political determinant of health, then and now. *Am J Public Health*. 2024;114(3):289–290.

Acceptance Date: December 23, 2023.

DOI: https://doi.org/10.2105/AJPH.2024.307579

CONFLICTS OF INTEREST

The author has no conflicts of interest to declare.

REFERENCES

1. Ransby B. *Ella Baker and the Black Freedom Movement.* Chapel Hill, NC: UNC Press; 2003.
2. US National Archives. John Lewis: March from Selma to Montgomery, "Bloody Sunday," 1965. Eyewitness: American Originals from the National Archives. Available at: https://www.archives.gov/exhibits/eyewitness/html.php?section=2. Accessed December 21, 2023.
3. History.Com Editors. Civil Rights Movement. History.Com website. Available at: https://www.history.com/topics/black-history/civil-rights-movement. Accessed December 21, 2023.
4. US Centers for Disease Control and Prevention. Social Determinants of Health at CDC. Available at: https://www.cdc.gov/about/sdoh/index.html. Updated December 8, 2022. Accessed December 22, 2023.
5. Navarro, V. What we mean by social determinants of health. *Int J Health Serv.* 2009;39(3):423-441. https://doi.org/10.2190/HS.39.3.A

Safeguarding Infant Lives: The Unappreciated Effects of Voting Rights Enforcement

Jesse H. Rhodes, PhD

ABOUT THE AUTHOR

Jesse H. Rhodes is with the Department of Political Science, University of Massachusetts Amherst.

See also Public Health Benefits of Voting Rights, Then and Now, pp. 289–308.

There is mounting evidence that increased voting and political participation are associated with improved public health, and the erection of barriers to voting can have deleterious public health consequences.[1,2] Yet over the past two decades, access to the ballot has become a contentious issue with strong partisan and racial overtones. Claiming (without evidence) that US elections are marred by widespread voter fraud, many Republicans, including former president Donald Trump, call for "election security" measures, such as voter ID laws, that make registration and voting more difficult.[3] Meanwhile, many Democrats contend that such measures aim to suppress the legitimate votes of people of color and advocate instead for policies like same-day registration and all-mail voting that expand ballot access.[4] This ideological divide has manifested at the state level, with Republican-controlled states imposing new barriers to voting and Democrat-controlled states adopting policies that enhance access to the ballot.[5] Recent research suggests that state partisan polarization in ballot accessibility may have contributed to interstate inequalities in public health outcomes in critical areas such as COVID-19 case and mortality rates.[6]

Partisan and geographic polarization in ballot access has been exacerbated by a conservative retrenchment in voting rights jurisprudence on the US Supreme Court. Since the 1970s, and accelerating between the 2000s and 2020s, the court's decisions have gradually eroded the Voting Rights Act (VRA), the most important federal voting rights law.[7] In its landmark decision in *Shelby County v Holder* (2013), the court invalidated a crucial provision requiring jurisdictions with histories of racial discrimination in voting to seek federal approval for proposed changes in their election laws.[8] The elimination of this preclearance requirement has made it easier for Republican governments in previously covered states to erect new barriers to voting that may disproportionately burden voters of color.[9]

Scholars are just beginning to grapple with the public health implications of the erosion of the federal government's capacity to enforce voting rights for communities of color. In this issue of *AJPH*, Rushovich et al. (p.300) shed light on this matter by appraising the historical impact of preclearance on infant mortality among African Americans and White Americans. Using data from 1959 to 1980, they applied difference-in-difference methods to examine pre- to post-VRA changes in deaths both in counties that were required to submit proposed changes in election laws and in comparable counties that were not subject to this requirement. What difference did preclearance have on infant mortality?

According to the authors, preclearance made the difference between life and death for thousands of African American infants between 1965 and 1980. African American infant deaths in preclearance-exposed counties decreased by 11.2 additional deaths per 1000 population of individuals younger than one year beyond the decrease experienced by unexposed counties between the pre-VRA period (1959–1965) and the immediate post-VRA period (1966–1970). This translates to 17.3% fewer African American infant deaths during this period than would have occurred in the absence of the federal preclearance requirement. The authors also reveal the longer-term impacts of preclearance by showing that African American infant deaths per 1000 population younger than one year in preclearance-exposed counties continued to decrease more swiftly relative to unexposed counties between 1971 and 1980. Notably, the beneficial effect of preclearance on infant survival was concentrated among African American infants, with no significant differences among Whites or the total population.

These findings provide compelling evidence that federal enforcement of the voting rights of African Americans goes beyond merely ensuring access to democracy for all. Rather, Rushovich et al.

suggest that federal enforcement established conditions under which African American citizens could advocate more effectively for the conditions necessary to sustain the lives of the most vulnerable members of their communities. This powerfully reinforces emerging research that documents the beneficial effect of preclearance on other outcomes in both the public and private sectors (i.e., access to federal funding, racially fair policing, and racially equitable wages) that are associated with improved health.[10–12]

Rushovich et al. quantify the benefits of preclearance, but they refrain from drawing any concrete policy recommendations from their findings. Why? Although we cannot know for sure, their reticence could be interpreted as a tacit acknowledgment that reinstatement of federal preclearance is all but impossible in the current political climate. Indeed, efforts spearheaded by congressional Democrats to reinstitute some form of federal preclearance in the wake of the *Shelby County* decision foundered because of lack of Republican support.[13]

Even so, we can still derive policy-relevant implications from their research. First, despite the high obstacles to success, public health leaders, voting rights activists, and others concerned with the well-being of marginalized communities should continue to advocate the reinstatement of preclearance at the national level. Second, and more immediately, these actors should use state voting rights policymaking to advance the public health interests of communities of color.

To date, six states—California, Washington, Oregon, Virginia, New York, and Connecticut—which collectively represent roughly 28% of the nation's population, have adopted state voting rights acts (SVRAs). Importantly, these state laws can go above the legal floor set by the federal VRA.[14,15] These acts, which differ in their specifics, are designed to grant communities of color more power to advance their interests in elections. For example, SVRAs in California, Washington, and Oregon make it easier for communities of color to challenge local representation schemes that may dilute their voting power; whereas New York's SVRA expands access for voters with limited English proficiency. Connecticut's and Virginia's SVRAs even feature state-level preclearance for communities that want to implement changes in their election laws.[16,17] The research of Rushovich et al., alongside previous work documenting the benefits of the VRA for communities of color, strongly implies that SVRAs may produce public health benefits for communities of color.

Admittedly, enacting voting rights protections state by state is an inadequate substitute for federal legislation. Given the high political bar to reinstatement of federal preclearance, however, public health advocates should take advantage of our system of federalism to make progress when and where they can. And states like California, which has had a SVRA since 2001, show that these laws can significantly improve representation for communities of color, with plausible downstream benefits for public health.[18] Although the work of Rushovich et al. focuses primarily on the historical impact of the federal VRA, it speaks in important ways to ongoing efforts to secure minority voting rights and improve public health outcomes for communities of color. AJPH

CORRESPONDENCE

Correspondence should be sent to Jesse H. Rhodes, Department of Political Science, University of Massachusetts, Amherst, 502 Thompson Tower, 200 Hicks Way, Amherst, MA 01003 (e-mail: jrhodes@polsci.umass.edu). Reprints can be ordered at http://www.ajph.org by clicking the "Reprints" link.

PUBLICATION INFORMATION

Full Citation: Rhodes JH. Safeguarding infant lives: the unappreciated effects of voting rights enforcement. *Am J Public Health*. 2024;114(3): 291–293.

Acceptance Date: December 19, 2023.

DOI: https://doi.org/10.2105/AJPH.2023.307566

ACKNOWLEDGMENTS

The author thanks the editors and the peer reviewers for their thoughtful comments. ChatGPT was used to recommend edits to improve the readability of the editorial.

CONFLICTS OF INTEREST

The author has no conflicts of interest to declare.

REFERENCES

1. Brown CL, Raza D, Pinto AD. Voting, health and interventions in healthcare settings: a scoping review. *Public Health Rev.* 2020;41:16. https://doi.org/10.1186/s40985-020-00133-6
2. Schraufnagel S. Voting restrictions and public health: an analysis of state variation 1996–2020. *State Local Gov Rev.* 2023;1:1–16. https://doi.org/10.1177/0160323X231202421
3. Eggers AC, Garro H, Grimmer J. No evidence for systematic voter fraud: a guide to statistical claims about the 2020 election. *Proc Natl Acad Sci USA.* 2021;118(45):e2103619118. https://doi.org/10.1073/pnas.2103619118
4. Hasen RL. *The Voting Wars: From Florida 2000 to the Next Election Meltdown.* New Haven, CT: Yale University Press; 2012.
5. Grumbach JM. Laboratories of democratic backsliding. *Am Polit Sci Rev.* 2023;117(3):967–984. https://doi.org/10.1017/S0003055422000934
6. Pabayo R, Grinshteyn E, Steele B, Cook DM, Muennig P, Liu SY. The relationship between voting restrictions and COVID-19 case and mortality rates between US counties. *PLoS One.* 2022;17(6): e0267738. https://doi.org/10.1371/journal.pone.0267738
7. Rhodes JH. *Ballot Blocked: The Political Erosion of the Voting Rights Act.* Stanford, CA: Stanford University Press; 2017.
8. US Supreme Court. *Shelby County v. Holder*, 570 US 529 (2013). Available at: https://supreme.justia.com/cases/federal/us/570/529. Accessed January 11, 2024.
9. Aneja AP, Avenancio-León CF. Disenfranchisement and economic inequality: downstream effects of *Shelby County v. Holder. AEA Pap Proc.* 2019;109: 161–165. https://doi.org/10.1257/pandp.20191085
10. Cascio EU, Washington E. Valuing the vote: the redistribution of voting rights and state funds following the Voting Rights Act of 1965. *Q J Econ.* 2014;129(1):379–433. https://doi.org/10.1093/qje/qjt028
11. Aneja A, Avenancio-León CF. The effect of political power on labor market inequality: evidence from the 1965 Voting Rights Act. October 2020. Available at: https://equitablegrowth.org/working-papers/the-effect-of-political-power-on-labor-market-inequality-evidence-from-the-1965-voting-rights-act. Accessed January 11, 2024.

12. Facchini G, Knight BG, Testa C. *The Franchise, Policing, and Race: Evidence From Arrests Data and the Voting Rights Act.* Cambridge, MA: National Bureau of Economic Research; 2020. NBER working paper 27463. https://doi.org/10.3386/w27463
13. Wang HL. Restoring the Voting Rights Act is still on this Alabama Democrat's agenda. September 19, 2023. Available at: https://www.npr.org/2023/09/19/1199617896/john-lewis-voting-rights-act-terri-sewell. Accessed January 11, 2024.
14. Legal Defense Fund. State voting rights acts: building a more inclusive democracy. 2023. Available at: https://www.naacpldf.org/ldf-mission/political-participation/state-voting-rights-protect-democracy. Accessed January 11, 2024.
15. Movement Advancement Project. State level voting rights acts. October 27, 2023. Available at: https://www.lgbtmap.org/democracy-maps/state_level_voting_rights_acts. Accessed January 11, 2024.
16. Sullivan C. Virginia's Voting Rights Act unpacked. *Democracy Docket.* November 9, 2021. Available at: https://www.democracydocket.com/analysis/virginias-voting-rights-act-unpacked. Accessed January 11, 2024.
17. Edison J. Gov. Ned Lamont signs CT voting rights act into law. *Ct Mirror.* June 12, 2023. Available at: https://ctmirror.org/2023/06/12/ct-voting-rights-act-law-elections. Accessed January 11, 2024.
18. Collingwood L, Long S. Can states promote minority representation? Assessing the effects of the California Voting Rights Act. *Urban Aff Rev.* 2021;57(3):731–762. https://doi.org/10.1177/1078087419896854

The Entrenched Erosion of Meaningful Participation in US Elections

Jennifer L. Pomeranz, JD, MPH

ABOUT THE AUTHORS

Jennifer L. Pomeranz is an associate professor in the Department of Public Health Policy and Management at the School of Global Public Health at New York University, New York, NY.

See also Public Health Benefits of Voting Rights, Then and Now, pp. 289–308.

The right to vote is a social determinant of health.[1] Voting is pivotal for community self-determination and to elect policymakers who will address structural inequalities and protect low-resourced and minoritized communities. In this issue, Rushovich et al. (p. 300) found that gaining the right to vote under the Voting Rights Act of 1965 (VRA) was associated with reduced Black infant deaths. Indeed, the Department of Justice referred to the VRA as "the single most effective piece of civil rights legislation passed by Congress."[2] Congress enacted the VRA to correct more than a century of disenfranchisement and prohibit states from restricting the right to vote in a discriminatory manner.

HISTORY OF VOTING RIGHTS IN THE UNITED STATES

The US Constitution provides states with the authority to regulate the time, place, and manner of holding elections. Under the auspices of this authority, states routinely proscribe who can vote by implementing restrictive requirements. At the founding of the United States, only White male landowners had the right to vote, followed by all White men by approximately 1860. Even though the passage of the 15th Amendment in 1870 ostensibly gave the right to vote to non-White men, and the passage of the 19th Amendment in 1920 gave the right to vote to women, states used their constitutional authority to enact restrictions that resulted in further disenfranchisement of predominantly non-White people. In 1924, the passage of the Indian Citizenship Act granted US citizenship to US-born Indigenous Americans, but this still did not provide Indigenous people the right to vote in many states.[3] It was not until decades later that state laws that overtly prohibited Indigenous Americans from voting were either struck down or repealed: Arizona and New Mexico in 1948, Utah in 1957, and North Dakota in 1958.[3] Furthermore, it was not until the passage of the VRA in 1965 that all Americans gained the undeniable right to vote.

The VRA's goal was to enforce the 15th Amendment's prohibition on denying the right to vote based on race or color. The US Supreme Court thereafter found that poll taxes and literacy tests were unconstitutional in 1966 and 1970, respectively. However, as discussed in Rushovich et al., in the 2013 case *Shelby County v Holder*, the Supreme Court struck down a primary provision of the VRA that required states with a history of racially motivated discriminatory practices to seek federal permission, known as "preclearance," before enacting any law related to voting.[4] The day the Supreme Court issued this decision, Texas implemented a new voter ID law that had previously been blocked through the preclearance process, and other states followed thereafter.[5]

MODERN VOTER SUPPRESSION

Thus, despite the VRA, states continue to enact laws that restrict the right to vote. These state laws generally include preemptive clauses that prohibit local governments and local elected officials from acting contrary to state law.[6] States use this tool for overt election interference, such as politically motivated gerrymandering,[7] and to hinder citizen-initiated ballot measures (e.g., referendums to repeal current laws[6]). Other states make it more difficult to vote. For example, Georgia closed 10% of its voting locations since *Shelby County v Holder*, despite a substantial increase in voter registration.[8] This resulted in hours-long wait times to vote in predominantly non-White communities.[8] Yet, in 2021, the state restricted relief workers' ability to provide water to prospective voters waiting on those long lines.[9]

States also continue to suppress Indigenous Americans' participation in elections. Indigenous people that live on reservations often rely on post office boxes for their mail.[3] Yet, some states do not allow the use of post office boxes to receive ballots, register to vote, or obtain government IDs needed to vote.[3] In 2018, North Dakota—which is home to five federally recognized tribes and an additional Indigenous community—enacted a voter ID law requiring the use of residential addresses and expressly excluding the use of post office boxes to qualify to vote.[3] North Dakota then redrew its districts in 2021, diluting two Indigenous American tribes' voting strength. In November 2023, a federal district court found this redistricting violated the VRA (*Turtle Mt Band of Chippewa Indians v Howe*, 2023 US Dist LEXIS 206894 [D ND November 17, 2023]).

Similarly, in 2022, North Carolina's highest state court struck down a state redistricting plan based on its finding of partisan gerrymandering. In response, the state went so far as to argue that state courts do not have judicial oversight over state election laws. The US Supreme Court disagreed and found that state rules concerning federal elections remain subject to the ordinary exercise of state judicial review (but it did not comment on the substance of the gerrymandering decision; *Moore v Harper*, 143 S Ct 2065 [2023]).

Of concern, however, are recent VRA cases. In October 2023, in *Petteway v Galveston County*, a federal district court in Texas found that Galveston County's redistricted map diluted the votes of Black and Latino voters in violation of—and "fundamentally inconsistent with"—the VRA.[7] In November 2023, the federal appellate court for the Fifth Circuit affirmed the district court's decision, but, thereafter, the Fifth Circuit stayed (or blocked) enforcement of the district court's decision and agreed to rehear the case *en banc*.[7] This means that Galveston County must use the redistricted map for its primary election in 2024 and that the Fifth Circuit may overturn the previous decisions, which would affirm the use of the redistricted map for future elections. Also in November 2023, in *Arkansas State Conference NAACP v Arkansas Board of Apportionment* (86 F 4th 1204 [8th Cir 2023]), the federal appellate court for the Eighth Circuit found that private plaintiffs (in that case the Arkansas NAACP and Arkansas Public Policy Panel) cannot sue to enforce the VRA, meaning that private plaintiffs who allege they have been denied the right to vote based on their race will have no legal recourse.

CAMPAIGN CONTRIBUTIONS

Beyond decisions chipping away at VRA protections, courts influence elections in additional ways that may undermine voting and public health. In the 2010 watershed case, *Citizens United v FEC*, the US Supreme Court found that corporations' campaign expenditures are a form of protected political speech under the First Amendment, meaning corporations have the same political speech rights as individuals.[10] Thereafter, in 2014, the Supreme Court struck down the Bipartisan Campaign Reform Act's aggregate contribution limits on campaign donors' ability to fund candidates, political parties, and Political Action Committees (PACs). The combination of these cases and additional court decisions led to the creation of Super PACs that can accept unlimited contributions from corporations, unions, and individuals, as well as "dark money" donations—those in which the source is not disclosed—estimated to be more than $2.6 billion since *Citizens United*.[11] Moreover, business interests—which often conflict with public health goals—made up $3.5 billion in federal political contributions alone for the 2022 election.[12] The erosion of transparent funding of election campaign speech is especially problematic in the context of protected speech itself: the First Amendment protects inaccurate, false, and deceptive political speech (e.g., misinformation campaigns).

POLICY IMPLICATIONS

As a result of the current system, campaigns are increasingly paid for by big money interests, and the time, place, and manner of elections are controlled by incumbent state administrations. Certain state voting restrictions favor keeping incumbents in office (e.g., partisan gerrymandering) and may result in fewer votes cast for policymakers that may challenge the status quo. This creates a cycle of disenfranchisement and low representation of minority interests among elected officials—and, thus, their political appointees, especially judges and justices whose role it is to interpret federal and state laws—solidifying incumbents' view of the law and constitutional protections.

Congress retains its constitutional authority to pass laws related to elections. Thus, Congress can preempt discriminatory state laws, fill the gap left by the 2013 gutting of the VRA, and reduce corporate influence in the wake of *Citizens United*. And there are members of Congress interested in these paths forward.[12,13] Although the current Supreme Court has indicated that it will not take into consideration social science research such as Rushovich et al. for its decisions, policymakers concerned with public health do consider such data in their decision-making. Thus, public health research should be disseminated to elected officials and voters to fuel support for transparent elections, address disparities, and undo decades of disenfranchisement in America. AJPH

CORRESPONDENCE

Correspondence should be sent to Jennifer L. Pomeranz, New York University, 708 Broadway, 7th Floor, New York, NY 10003 (e-mail: jlp284@nyu.edu). Reprints can be ordered at http://www.ajph.org by clicking the "Reprints" link.

PUBLICATION INFORMATION

Full Citation: Pomeranz JL. The entrenched erosion of meaningful participation in US elections. *Am J Public Health*. 2024;114(3):294–296.

Acceptance Date: December 19, 2023.

DOI: https://doi.org/10.2105/AJPH.2023.307567

ACKNOWLEDGMENTS

The author relied on the Library of Congress's website, The Right to Vote, (https://www.loc.gov/classroom-materials/elections/right-to-vote) for the history of voting rights in the United States.

CONFLICTS OF INTEREST

The author has no conflicts of interest to disclose.

REFERENCES

1. Ganguly A, Morelli D, Bhavan KP. Voting as a social determinant of health: leveraging health systems to increase access to voting. *NEJM Catalyst*. January 26, 2023. Available at: https://catalyst.nejm.org/doi/full/10.1056/CAT.22.0368. Accessed December 12, 2023.
2. US Department of Justice, Civil Rights Division. Introduction to federal voting rights laws. Available at: https://www.justice.gov/crt/introduction-federal-voting-rights-laws-0. Accessed December 12, 2023.
3. Ferguson-Bohnee P. How the Native American vote continues to be suppressed. American Bar Association. February 9, 2020. Available at: https://www.americanbar.org/groups/crsj/publications/human_rights_magazine_home/voting-rights/how-the-native-american-vote-continues-to-be-suppressed. Accessed December 12, 2023.
4. *Shelby County v Holder*, 570 US 529 (2013).
5. Effects of *Shelby County v Holder* on the Voting Rights Act. Brennan Center for Justice. June 21, 2023. Available at: https://www.brennancenter.org/our-work/research-reports/effects-shelby-county-v-holder-voting-rights-act. Accessed December 12, 2023.
6. Editorial Board. States are silencing the will of millions of voters. *New York Times*. June 3, 2023. Available at: https://www.nytimes.com/2023/06/03/opinion/texas-preemption-bill.html. Accessed December 12, 2023.
7. *Petteway v Galveston Cnty*, 2023 US Dist LEXIS 183978 (SD Tex October 13, 2023); *aff'd, Petteway v Galveston Cnty*, 86 F 4th 214 (5th Cir 2023); *rehearing en banc granted, opinion vacated, Petteway v Galveston Cnty*, 87 F 4th 721 (5th Cir 2023).
8. Fowler S. Why do nonwhite Georgia voters have to wait in line for hours? Too few polling places. *NPR*. October 17, 2020. Available at: https://www.npr.org/2020/10/17/924527679/why-do-nonwhite-georgia-voters-have-to-wait-in-line-for-hours-too-few-polling-pl. Accessed December 12, 2023.
9. *Sixth Dist of the African Methodist Episcopal Church v Kemp* (in re Ga. Senate Bill 202), 2023 US Dist LEXIS 144919 (ND Ga 2023).
10. *Citizens United v FEC*, 558 US 310 (2010).
11. Massoglia A. "Dark money" groups have poured billions into federal elections since the Supreme Court's 2010 Citizens United decision. *OpenSecrets*. January 24, 2023. Available at: https://www.opensecrets.org/news/2023/01/dark-money-groups-have-poured-billions-into-federal-elections-since-the-supreme-courts-2010-citizens-united-decision. Accessed December 12, 2023.
12. Giorno T. Business interests spent $3.5 billion on federal political contributions during the 2022 cycle. OpenSecrets. January 27, 2023. Available at: https://www.opensecrets.org/news/2023/01/business-interests-spent-3-5-billion-on-federal-political-contributions-during-the-2022-cycle. Accessed December 12, 2023.
13. Deutsch J. Congress has another chance to restore the Voting Rights Act. Campaign Legal Center. September 18, 2023 Available at: https://campaignlegal.org/update/congress-has-another-chance-restore-voting-rights-act. Accessed December 12, 2023.

Building Power, Advancing Health Equity: Insights From Voting and Beyond

Anna K. Hing, PhD, MPH

ABOUT THE AUTHOR

Anna K. Hing is with the Center for Antiracism Research for Health Equity and the Division of Health Policy and Management, University of Minnesota, Minneapolis.

See also Public Health Benefits of Voting Rights, Then and Now, pp. 289–308.

In their impactful work, Rushovich et al. (p. 300) investigate the effects of passing the US Voting Rights Act in 1965 on population health inequities. The Voting Rights Act was created to prevent racial discrimination at the polls, and the provision of voting rights led to dramatic improvements in health for Black, but not White, infants. This instructive research pushes us to consider both social and political determinants of health and to interrogate the role of racism in such analyses. Voting is a critical, albeit often overlooked, factor influencing population health. Although the field of public health is beginning to study voting as a determinant of health, it must also move further upstream to consider, more broadly, how power creates and maintains health inequities.

VOTING RIGHTS AND HEALTH

Rushovich et al. argue that the Voting Rights Act protected the right to vote and resulted in improvements in political power and social determinants of health. With the *Shelby County v Holder* decision in 2013, preclearance was invalidated, removing the requirement that states with a history of discrimination at the polls obtain federal approval before making changes to voting policies. Since the court's decision a decade ago, 29 states have passed 94 restrictive voting laws; 11 of those states were formerly covered by the preclearance mandate.[1] Consequently, the disparity in voter turnout between White and Black voters has increased.[1]

Given that the protection of voting rights is associated with improved health, as Rushovich et al. show, we should anticipate that decisions such as *Shelby County v Holder* and subsequent attacks on voting rights will be associated with poorer health.[2] There are many conceptual pathways through which voting affects health,[3] and public health researchers are beginning to investigate these mechanisms. For example, Pabayo et al. have linked state-level voting restrictions using the Cost of Voting Index with access to health insurance[4] and COVID-19 case and mortality rates,[5] showing that restrictions in voting rights are negatively associated with health.

STRUCTURAL RACISM IN VOTING ANALYSES

In the United States, voting has been deployed and protected as a way to uphold White supremacy and concentrate power along racial lines.[3] When the United States was founded, only White, landowning men could vote. Even after the passing of the Fifteenth Amendment, which expanded the vote to men of any race, poll taxes and literacy tests prevented Black men and men from other racialized groups from voting. Contemporary voting laws follow in this tradition; although they may appear race neutral, felony disenfranchisement laws and voter identification laws disproportionately exclude voters racialized as Black.[6] Other forms of racist disenfranchisement include purging voter rolls, closing polling places in predominantly Black and Brown neighborhoods, reducing early voting days, and restricting mail-in voting. Furthermore, the electoral college[7] and Senate representation[8] have been shown to dilute the voting power of Black voters. By tracing the history of the discrimination that the Voting Rights Act was trying to protect against, we can clearly situate voter suppression as a form of structural racism.[3]

Structural racism operates as a system of interwoven institutions.[9] Voting restrictions are an especially insidious domain of structural racism, as they form a critical pathway to perpetuate this system by reaching across institutions. This "inter-institutional connection" is necessary to maintain structural White supremacy.[9(p294)] By building rules to uphold White supremacy in electoral processes—one place where this

AJPH March 2024, Vol. 114, No. 3

ideology could be challenged and antiracist policies realized—the durability of structural racism is ensured. Thus, challenges to structural racism must come from building alternative forms of power and determining how to redistribute power in these institutions.

POWER AND HEALTH EQUITY

Beyond voting, we must consider power more broadly and interrogate how power operates as a fundamental determinant of health.[10] Restrictions to voting that target racialized voters are fundamentally about power: who can wield power and what that power can be used to achieve. White supremacy seeks to concentrate power among those racialized as White, and voting restrictions are one part of the disempowerment process.

The US democratic system is founded on the ideology of White supremacy, yet we are told to use this system to enact change that will yield health equity. Because of its racist origins, the status quo of racial inequity can never be fully challenged. As writer and activist Audre Lorde said, the master's tools will never dismantle the master's house. Voting is a domesticated form of power: it is nonthreatening, controlled, subjugated. The influence of voting exists only in the electoral system, and although voting is still a critical action for making peoples' voices heard, those voices can be silenced. Voting in an unjust system cannot bring about true change. Therefore, to move toward health equity, public health must consider alternative forms of power beyond voting, how those alternatives can be wielded to improve health, and what the potential health effects of participating in, building, and realizing those alternate forms of power can be.

The redistribution of power to historically marginalized and racialized groups is inherently antiracist. Racial inequities exist not because of genetics or chance but because they are created. Race and racism are socially constructed, and the hierarchies of power and distribution of resources we observe are a result of this process. To alter the inequitable distribution of resources, we need to critically reconceptualize who has power and reconsider which types of power are judged legitimate. It was only through the direct action of the civil rights movement, the women's suffrage movement, and other campaigns that the vote has been expanded, but we still see that one person does not equal one vote.[11]

RENEGOTIATING POWER WITH DIRECT ACTION

As the field of public health moves to consider how power influences health, we should distinguish between individual and collective power and consider the levels at which we measure power. Voting analyses commonly use state-level measures, but this masks critical processes occurring at more local levels. The distribution of power varies by geographic location—as do efforts to suppress that power. Polling place closures in predominantly Black neighborhoods require people to travel farther and have led to wait times of hours,[12] but this disparity may not be captured with a state-level analysis. Rather, struggles for power and power redistribution are often local. For example, tenant organizing is one method of reclaiming power.[10] This type of organizing happens in neighborhoods and cities, not at the state level, and is a reaction to a very specific nexus of local conditions.

In addition to tenant strikes, labor strikes have produced dramatic shifts in power back to workers. By the end of October 2023, 354 strikes by 492 000 workers were recorded for 2023, which was four times the number of people in the same period in 2022 and included workers from the United Auto Workers, Screen Actors Guild–American Federation of Television and Radio Artists, and Kaiser Permanente.[13] These strikes introduced people to direct action and organizing and showed that collective action can yield improvements in known social determinants of health, including income and working conditions. Furthermore, workers at major corporations, including Amazon and Starbucks, are unionizing. Labor strikes, unionizing, protests, and other organizing efforts that build power can act as tools to realize health equity.

As researchers in public health, we should work with those who study movement building, collective action, labor, and labor organizing to better understand the forces at play and how these movements shape social conditions and health. None of this research can be conducted without centering the people doing this work on the ground. If public health is truly concerned with understanding power, the field must move toward redistributing power in its own knowledge production processes, which so often reinforce power inequities between the academy and community rather than breaking them down.

CONCLUSIONS

Public health cannot achieve health equity without working to reform the electoral system. Our individual and community-level interventions become obsolete if courts selected by the president can take away the right to abortion or limit other human rights. But voting is just one form of power. Public health should prioritize supporting grassroots organizing efforts that build power and improve health. As Michener states, "achieving health justice requires *both* building power among those who are most deeply affected (corporeally and materially) by health inequity *and* breaking the power of those who are accruing (economic and political) gains from the status quo of health inequity."[14(p657; emphasis in original)] In studying voting, we cannot forget that we are studying power, how it is stratified, and how inequities in power yield inequities in health. The redistribution of power is necessary for achieving health equity.

AJPH

CORRESPONDENCE

Correspondence should be sent to Anna K. Hing, 2001 Plymouth Ave N, Suite 106, Minneapolis, MN 55411 (e-mail: hing0013@umn.edu). Reprints can be ordered at http://www.ajph.org by clicking the "Reprints" link.

PUBLICATION INFORMATION

Full Citation: Hing AK. Building power, advancing health equity: insights from voting and beyond. *Am J Public Health*. 2024;114(3):297–299.

Acceptance Date: December 21, 2023.

DOI: https://doi.org/10.2105/AJPH.2024.307578

CONFLICTS OF INTEREST

The author has no conflicts of interest to declare.

REFERENCES

1. Singh J, Carter S. States have added nearly 100 restrictive laws since SCOTUS gutted the Voting Rights Act 10 years ago. June 23, 2023. Available at: https://www.brennancenter.org/our-work/analysis-opinion/states-have-added-nearly-100-restrictive-laws-scotus-gutted-voting-rights. Accessed December 15, 2023.
2. Hing AK. Suppressing the vote, suppressing future voters: a multilevel analysis of voter suppression and Black–White disparities in life expectancy and infant outcomes. Available at: https://www.proquest.com/docview/2584355805?pq-origsite=gscholar&fromopenview=true&sourcetype=Dissertations%20&%20Theses. Accessed January 16, 2024.
3. Hing AK. The right to vote, the right to health: voter suppression as a determinant of racial health disparities. *J Health Dispar Res Pract.* 2018;12(6):article 5. Available at: https://digitalscholarship.unlv.edu/jhdrp/vol12/iss6/5. Accessed January 16, 2024.
4. Pabayo R, Liu SY, Grinshteyn E, Cook DM, Muennig P. Barriers to voting and access to health insurance among US adults: a cross-sectional study. *Lancet Reg Health Am.* 2021;2:100026. https://doi.org/10.1016/j.lana.2021.100026
5. Pabayo R, Grinshteyn E, Steele B, Cook DM, Muennig P, Liu SY. The relationship between voting restrictions and COVID-19 case and mortality rates between US counties. *PLoS ONE.* 2022;17(6):e0267738. https://doi.org/10.1371/journal.pone.0267738
6. Behrens A, Uggen C, Manza J. Ballot manipulation and the "menace of Negro domination": racial threat and felon disenfranchisement in the United States, 1850–2002. *Am J Sociol.* 2003;109(3):559–605. https://doi.org/10.1086/378647
7. Codrington WU III. The electoral college's racist origins. April 1, 2020. Available at: https://www.brennancenter.org/our-work/analysis-opinion/electoral-colleges-racist-origins. Accessed December 15, 2023.
8. Malhotra N, Raso C. Racial representation and U.S. Senate apportionment. *Soc Sci Q.* 2007;88(4):1038–1048. https://doi.org/10.1111/j.1540-6237.2007.00517.x
9. Gee GC, Hicken MT. Structural racism: the rules and relations of inequity. *Ethn Dis.* 2021;31(suppl 1):293–300. https://doi.org/10.18865/ed.31.S1.293
10. Michener J. Racism, power, and health equity: the case of tenant organizing. *Health Aff (Millwood).* 2023;42(10):1318–1324. https://doi.org/10.1377/hlthaff.2023.00509
11. Anderson C. *One Person, No Vote: How Voter Suppression Is Destroying Our Democracy.* London, UK: Bloomsbury Publishing; 2018.
12. Fowler S. Why do nonwhite Georgia voters have to wait in line for hours? Too few polling places. October 17, 2020. Available at: https://www.npr.org/2020/10/17/924527679/why-do-nonwhite-georgia-voters-have-to-wait-in-line-for-hours-too-few-polling-pl. Accessed December 15, 2023.
13. Bronfenbrenner K. For labor unions, 2023 was the year of the strike—and big victories. *Wall Street Journal.* December 4, 2023. Available at: https://www.wsj.com/business/unions-workers-2023-strikes-companies-da09de12. Accessed December 15, 2023.
14. Michener J. Health justice through the lens of power. *J Law Med Ethics.* 2022;50(4):656–662. https://doi.org/10.1017/jme.2023.5

1965 US Voting Rights Act Impact on Black and Black Versus White Infant Death Rates in Jim Crow States, 1959–1980 and 2017–2021

Tamara Rushovich, MPH, Rachel C. Nethery, PhD, Ariel White, PhD, and Nancy Krieger, PhD

See also Public Health Benefits of Voting Rights, Then and Now, pp. 289–299.

Objectives. To investigate the impact of the US Voting Rights Act (VRA) of 1965 on Black and Black versus White infant deaths in Jim Crow states.

Methods. Using data from 1959 to 1980 and 2017 to 2021, we applied difference-in-differences methods to quantify differential pre–post VRA changes in infant deaths in VRA-exposed versus unexposed counties, controlling for population size and social, economic, and health system characteristics. VRA-exposed counties, identified by Section 4, were subject to government interventions to remove existing racist voter suppression policies.

Results. Black infant deaths in VRA-exposed counties decreased by an average of 11.4 (95% confidence interval [CI] = 1.7, 21.0) additional deaths beyond the decrease experienced by unexposed counties between the pre-VRA period (1959–1965) and the post-VRA period (1966–1970). This translates to 6703 (95% CI = 999.6, 12 348) or 17.5% (95% CI = 3.1%, 28.1%) fewer deaths than would have been experienced in the absence of the VRA. The equivalent differential changes were not significant among the White or total population.

Conclusions. Passage of the VRA led to pronounced reductions in Black infant deaths in Southern counties subject to government intervention because these counties had particularly egregious voter suppression practices. (*Am J Public Health*. 2024;114(3):300–308. https://doi.org/10.2105/AJPH.2023.307518)

AJPH March 2024, Vol. 114, No. 3

In 2013, the US Supreme Court ruled in *Shelby County v Holder* that Section 4 of the Voting Rights Act of 1965 (VRA) was unconstitutional. As a result, jurisdictions with a history of discriminatory voting practices no longer needed federal approval prior to making changes to their voting procedures.[1] Amid this backdrop, public health studies began to focus more on how political context affects health.[2,3]

Simultaneously, public health research documenting the harms of racism has increased drastically in recent years.[4] Voter suppression is 1 mechanism by which structural racism operates to systematically prevent Black and other populations of color from participating in American democracy. After the end of the Civil War, Congress passed the 13th, 14th, and 15th amendments to the US Constitution in 1865, 1868, and 1870, respectively. These amendments abolished slavery, established citizenship, and established voting rights for Black men; however, by the 1880s Black men were effectively prevented from voting through Jim Crow laws—including poll taxes and literacy tests—that were in effect in 21 US states and the District of Columbia[5,6] When the VRA was passed in 1965, the use of any "device," such as a literacy test, in voter registration became illegal and jurisdictions with a history of discriminatory voting practices were required to receive federal approval prior to altering their voting practices.[7]

It is well documented that the VRA increased Black voter turnout, increased the number of Black elected officials, and influenced the voting decisions of representatives.[8–10] Existing studies have explored the social and economic impacts of the VRA and showed additional increases in state fund transfers,[11] decreases in the Black–White wage gap,[12] and decreases in Black arrest rates[13] in areas most affected by the VRA. These improvements in the social and economic conditions are also known determinants of health.[14] Several studies have shown that higher voter participation is associated with better health.[15–17] To date, however, there are no studies directly investigating the health impacts of the VRA.

Informed by the ecosocial theory of disease distribution,[18] which posits that population distributions of health and health inequities reflect embodied political, economic, social, and material contexts, the primary objectives of this study were to investigate the effect of US government intervention to remove existing racist voter suppression policies as specified by the VRA on infant deaths overall, Black infant deaths, and racialized inequities in infant deaths in former Jim Crow states. Additionally, we used data from 2017 to 2021 to investigate potential remaining footprints of the VRA in contemporary infant mortality rates.

METHODS

Our primary analysis used US vital statistics data on county-level infant deaths[19] and US census data on county population and sociodemographic characteristics for the years 1959 to 1980.[20,21] We compared infant deaths during the pre-VRA period (1959–1965) to infant deaths in 3 post-VRA periods (1966–1970, 1971–1975, and 1976–1980) to quantify short-, intermediate-, and long-term effects. We also conducted a secondary exploratory analysis of long-term trends using an additional post-VRA period of 2017 to 2021.[22]

The study population was restricted to counties within states that had Jim Crow laws, and thereby shared a common history of legal racialized segregation. Jim Crow states were defined as having a documented law or ordinance enforcing racial discrimination as identified in *States' Laws on Race and Color*, published in 1950 by Pauli Murray.[6] Our analysis investigated variation within the Jim Crow context to test whether counties with particularly egregious voter suppression histories (which therefore met the criteria specified in Section 4 of the VRA) experienced a disproportionate reduction in infant deaths after having been subject to government intervention specified by the VRA.

Exposure

The entire United States was subject to the broad regulations of the VRA. In this study, exposure was defined at the county level as being covered by Section 4 of the VRA in 1965, 1970, or both years, and therefore subject to the requirements specified in Section 5 of the VRA (for more details, see Figure 1 and parts A, B, and C of the Appendix, available as a supplement to the online version of this article at http://www.ajph.org). Section 4 designated any jurisdiction that utilized a "device" (e.g., a literacy test) to determine voter eligibility and had voter registration or turnout under 50% for the 1964 election. Section 5 specified the removal of all "devices" and required preclearance (i.e., federal approval) of any policy changes relating to voting practices for all counties that met the coverage formula in Section 4.[7] The VRA coverage formula criteria were updated in 1970 and expanded in 1975 to include language-based voting barriers. By these criteria, among the 21 Jim Crow states plus the District of Columbia, 587 counties located in 8 states were VRA-covered and 1113 counties in 16 states were not VRA-covered.

Outcome

The outcome for this study was infant death, defined as death from any cause prior to age 1 year, which is a common measure of population health as it is sensitive to social and economic living conditions throughout pregnancy and during the infant's first year of life.[23–25] We conducted separate analyses using all infant deaths and infant deaths stratified by racialized group.

County-level covariates for 1960 comprised the Index of Concentration at the Extremes for income,[26] the percentage of the population that was Black, population density, unemployment rate, and presence of a desegregated hospital; see technical definitions in the part E of the Appendix.

Statistical Analysis

First, we calculated descriptive statistics using infant death rates per 1000 population of individuals aged younger than 1 year for the study population over the study period. Next, we used a series of difference-in-differences (DID) linear regression models to estimate the effect of the VRA on infant deaths. We used a linear model instead of the commonly used log-linear model for count or rate outcomes to preserve the requisite parallel trends assumption for the DID. We used infant death counts

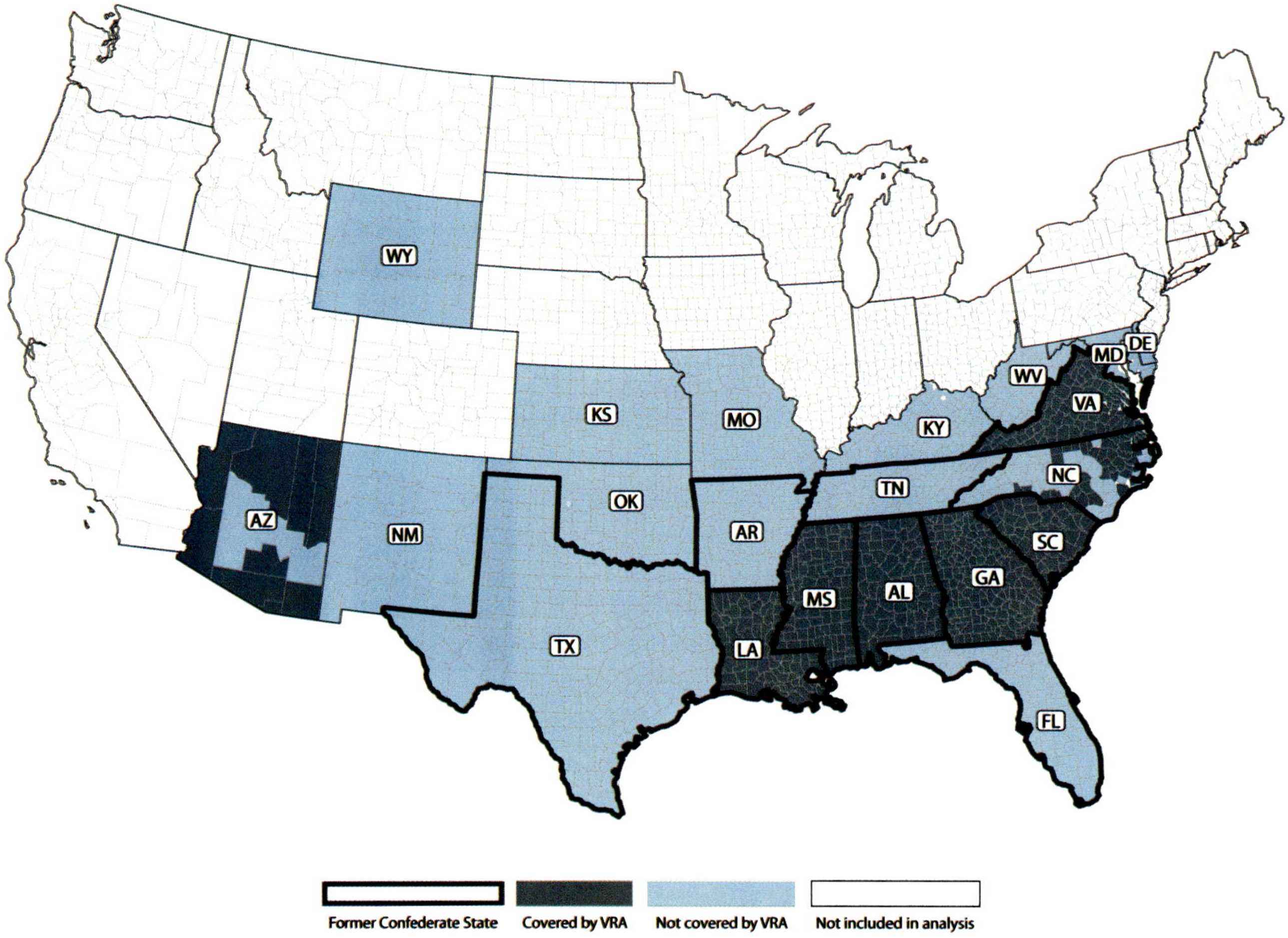

FIGURE 1— Voting Rights Act of 1965 (VRA) Coverage by County Among Former Jim Crow States: United States, 1965 and 1970

as the outcome, with model-based adjustment for population size, instead of directly modeling rate outcomes, to allow the model to better distinguish between a zero count of death in strata with small population versus a zero count of death in a strata with a large population at low risk of the outcome.[27]

The following DID model was used to estimate the effect of the VRA on overall infant deaths, aggregated across racialized groups:

$$E(Y) = \beta_0 + \beta_1 Post + \beta_2 VRA * Post + \beta_3 Pop + \alpha_{state} + \boldsymbol{\delta}'\mathbf{X} \quad (1)$$

The units of analysis are county-time periods. County-year strata are aggregated to the pre-VRA time period (1959–1965), 3 temporally proximal post-VRA time periods (1966–1970, 1971–1975, and 1976–1980), and the 2017–2021 time period, and we fit separate models for each post-VRA time period. The outcome (Y) is the count of infant deaths for each county-time period. Covariates comprised (1) the main effect for time period (β_1), (2) population size for each county-time period (β_3), (3) fixed effects for state (α_{state}), and (4) a vector of county sociodemographic characteristics in 1960 ($\boldsymbol{\delta}$). Note that an explicit VRA main effect term was omitted from the model because of collinearity with the state fixed effects, which were included to control for all state-level time-invariant characteristics (e.g., state-level policies). In this model, β_2, the coefficient for the interaction term between the indicator variable for being covered by the VRA and an indicator for post-VRA time period, is the primary parameter of interest and can be interpreted as the on-average additional decrease in infant deaths from the pre-VRA to the post-VRA period in covered counties compared with noncovered counties (referred to as "the effect").

We used an analogous model specification for the racialized group-specific models—that is, we fit models with the same structure but using as the outcome infant death counts in a single racialized group (for each county-time period) and substituting the racialized group-specific population size for the total population size. For formal comparisons and tests for differences in the additional effect of the VRA on Black deaths compared with White deaths, we fit an additional analogous triple DID model to the racialized group-stratified data. This model is specified in more detail in part F of the Appendix. We obtained cluster and heteroskedastic-robust standard errors, which account for clustering at the state level, for all models.

Assumptions for Difference-in-Differences

The causal interpretation of the DID estimator relies on the assumption of parallel trends, meaning that the trend in the outcome for the exposed group (i.e., covered by the VRA) would have been parallel to the outcome in the unexposed group in the post-VRA period had the intervention (i.e., VRA) not occurred, conditional on covariates adjusted for in the model. Although it was not possible to evaluate this counterfactual scenario directly, we assessed plausibility by empirically testing for parallel trends in infant deaths during the pre-VRA period. We used both data visualization and statistical tests to identify any differential pre-VRA trends in infant deaths in covered and noncovered counties. We plotted the trend in yearly observed infant deaths by coverage status and racialized group (aggregated across counties) during the period prior to the passage of the VRA. We fit the model $E(Y)=\gamma_0+\gamma_1 year+\gamma_2 year*VRA+\gamma_3 Pop+\rho_{state}+\boldsymbol{\eta}'\mathbf{X}$ to pre-VRA infant death data (with county-years as the unit of analysis) to test for parallel trends over time between covered and noncovered counties prior to VRA implementation. The parameter of interest is γ_2 , which describes the differential change in infant deaths over time in covered compared with noncovered counties, controlling for county population and state fixed effects. We used the same model specifications, but with added interaction terms between racialized group and each variable (the parameter of interest was from the triple interaction term between *racialized group * year * VRA*), to test for parallel trends in the Black–White disparity in infant deaths during the pre-VRA period.

Classification of Racialized Groups

Our analysis focused on the US Black and White populations; see part D of the Appendix for the methods we used to construct these social groups using the racialized categories available in the mortality data and census counts for each time period.

Because the VRA primarily changed voting access for Black Americans, using data for "non-White" individuals instead of only Black individuals could introduce bias. To investigate potential bias, we conducted a sensitivity analyses, in which the models used in the main analysis (specified in the Statistical Analysis section) were repeated using a version of the data set that used the classifications "White" and "non-White" for 1959 to 1969 and "White" and "Black" for 1970 to 1980 when the more granular data were available. For more detail, see part D of the Appendix.

Robustness Analyses

We also conducted the DID analyses within the former Confederate states, which is a subset of the Jim Crow polity. This subset was of interest because all the states had a shared history of enslavement of Black people as well as Jim Crow laws. To investigate the effect of the VRA within a single state, and thus fully controlling for state-level policies, we ran the same models only within North Carolina, 1 of 2 states that had within-state and between-county variation in VRA coverage status.

RESULTS

In former Jim Crow states, there were 588 VRA-covered counties and 1112 noncovered counties (Figure 1). In 1960, the VRA-covered versus noncovered counties had a higher percentage of Black residents, lower educational attainment, lower median family income, higher population density, more extreme economic segregation, and fewer desegregated hospitals (Table A, available as a supplement to the online version of this article at http://www.ajph.org). In the pre-VRA period (1959–1965), the rate of infant deaths was 34.3 per 1000 population in covered counties and 28.9 in noncovered counties; in 1976, these rates respectively equaled 16.8 and 14.9 per 1000. Among Black Americans, the infant death rate in 1959 to 1965 was 51.9 in covered counties and 48.1 in noncovered counties; in 1976 to 1980, these rates were respectively 24.9 and 20.1 per 1000 population. In 2017 to 2021, these rates were one fifth the 1959–1965 rates (Table 1; Figure B, available as a supplement to the online version of this article at http://www.ajph.org).

Assumptions for Difference-in-Differences

The estimate of the coefficient for *year * VRA* from the model testing for parallel trends in Black infant deaths during the pre-VRA period was

TABLE 1— Aggregate Infant Mortality Rates per 1000 Children Younger than 1 Year for Counties Covered vs Not Covered by the Voting Rights Act of 1965 (VRA) in Former Jim Crow States: United States, 1959–1980 and 2017–2021

	Covered by VRA		Not Covered by VRA	
	Count	Rate per 1000 (95% CI)	Count	Rate per 1000 (95% CI)
Total population				
Pre-VRA: 1959–1965	121 104	34.25 (34.25, 34.25)	188 881	28.92 (28.92, 28.92)
Post-VRA: 1966–1970	61 583	27.23 (27.23, 27.23)	98 011	23.22 (23.22, 23.22)
Post-VRA: 1971–1975	45 608	21.03 (21.03, 21.03)	76 652	18.53 (18.53, 18.53)
Post-VRA: 1976–1980	36 383	16.79 (16.79, 16.79)	63 250	14.87 (14.87, 14.87)
Post-VRA: 2017–2021	16 676	7.01 (7.01, 7.01)	33 822	5.96 (5.96, 5.97)
Black infant deaths				
Pre-VRA: 1959–1965	65 998	51.93 (51.93, 51.93)	53 911	48.13 (48.13, 48.13)
Post-VRA: 1966–1970	31 617	41.62 (41.62, 41.62)	28 041	38.11 (38.11, 38.11)
Post-VRA: 1971–1975	22 134	30.40 (30.40, 30.340)	20 944	26.43 (26.43, 26.43)
Post-VRA: 1976–1980	18 948	24.90 (24.90, 24.90)	18 566	20.06 (20.06, 20.06)
Post-VRA: 2017–2021	9 023	10.42 (10.42, 10.42)	11 645	9.56 (9.56, 9.56)
White infant deaths				
Pre-VRA: 1959–1965	55 106	24.33 (24.33, 24.33)	134 970	24.94 (24.94, 24.94)
Post-VRA: 1966–1970	29 966	19.95 (19.95, 19.95)	69 970	20.07 (20.07, 20.07)
Post-VRA: 1971–1975	23 474	16.30 (16.30, 16.30)	55 708	16.66 (16.66, 16.66)
Post-VRA: 1976–1980	17 435	12.40 (12.40, 12.40)	44 684	13.43 (13.43, 13.43)
Post-VRA: 2017–2021	7 653	5.06 (5.06, 5.06)	22 177	4.98 (4.98, 4.98)

Note. CI = confidence interval. Covered by VRA: AL, GA, LA, MS, SC, VA, 39 counties in NC, 9 counties in AZ. Not covered by VRA: AR, DE, DC, FL, KS, KY, MD, MO, NM, OK, TN, TX, WV, WY, 61 counties in NC, 5 counties in AZ.

AJPH March 2024, Vol. 114, No. 3

0.0000027 (95% confidence interval [CI] = −0.00360, 0.00361; P = .9), indicating that the annual trend in infant deaths over time was not significantly different for covered compared with noncovered counties. The estimate of the coefficient for *year* ∗ *VRA* ∗ *racialized group* was −0.13 (95% CI = −0.34, 0.074; P = .18). This provided evidence to support the main assumption of parallel trends in the pre-VRA period of the DID estimator (Figure 2; Figures A and C, available as a supplement to the online version of this article at http://www.ajph.org).

Difference-in-Differences Regression Results

The results from the DID regression model for the total population counts of infant deaths showed that overall infant deaths decreased between the pre-VRA period and all 3 post-VRA periods. In noncovered counties, the average change in infant deaths from the pre-VRA period to the 1966–1970 post-VRA period was −28.8 (95% CI = −40.4, −17.1) deaths per county (−49.2 [95% CI = −68.0, −30.4] and −65.5 [95% CI = −89.9, −41.1]) in the 1971–1975 and 1976–1980 post-VRA periods, respectively). In covered counties, the average additional change in infant deaths above and beyond that experienced in noncovered counties (the VRA effect) from the pre-VRA period to the 1966–1970 post-VRA period was −13.1 (95% CI = −29.3, 3.2) deaths per county (−18.2 [95% CI = −43.5, 7.1] and −19.9 [95% CI = −51.0, 11.3] in the 1971–1975 and 1976–1980 post-VRA periods, respectively). However, none of these effects were statistically significant (Table 2; Table B, available as a supplement to the online version of this article at http://www.ajph.org).

The racialized group-specific DID models showed that the mean change in Black infant deaths from the pre-VRA period to the 1966–1970 post-VRA period in noncovered counties was −8.9 (95% CI = −14.1, −3.8) deaths per county (and −18.8 [95% CI = −28.2, −9.4] and −26.6 [95% CI = −40.3, −13.0] in the 1971–1975 and 1976–1980 post-VRA periods, respectively; Table 2 and Table C, available as a supplement to the online version of this article at http://www.ajph.org). Moreover, in covered counties the mean additional change in Black

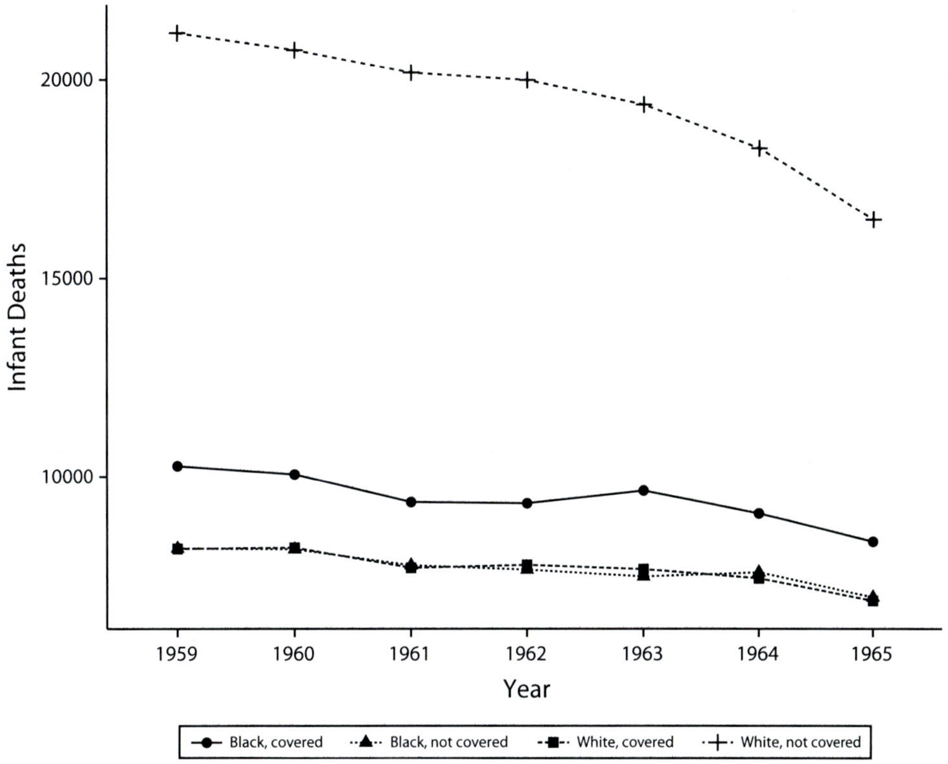

FIGURE 2— Trends in Infant Deaths Prior to the Voting Rights Act of 1965 (VRA) in Former Jim Crow States: United States, 1959–1965

Note. The $\gamma_2 year * VRA$ coefficient value is 0.00058 (SE = 0.0014, P = .74) for Black infant deaths and 0.0064 (SE = 0.00051, P = .42) for White infant deaths. The coefficient values were calculated from the regression model: $E(Y) = \gamma_0 + \gamma_1 year + \gamma_2 year * VRA + \gamma_3 Pop + \rho_{state} + \boldsymbol{\eta}' \boldsymbol{X}$, where X is a vector of covariates that include the Index of Concentration at the Extremes for income, the percentage of the county population that was Black, county population density, county unemployment rate, and presence of a desegregated hospital. Covered by VRA: AL, GA, LA, MS, SC, VA, 39 counties in NC, 9 counties in AZ. Not covered by VRA: AR, DE, DC, FL, KS, KY, MD, MO, NM, OK, TN, TX, WV, WY, 61 counties in NC, 5 counties in AZ.

infant deaths (the VRA effect) from the pre-VRA period to the 1966–1970 post-VRA period was −11.4 (95% CI = −21.0, −1.7) deaths per county (−18.1 [95% CI = −34.4, −1.9] and −21.6 [95% CI = −42.4, −0.9] in the 1971–1975 and 1976–1980 post-VRA periods, respectively). These effects were statistically significant for all time periods. This equated to an estimated 6703 (95% CI = 999.6, 12 348) fewer Black infant deaths in the 1966–1970 post-VRA period or a 17.5% (95% CI = 3.1%, 38.1%) reduction. White infant deaths also decreased from the pre- to the post-VRA period in both covered and noncovered counties, but the VRA effect was not statistically significant in the White population (Table 2; Table D, available as a supplement to the online version of this article at http://www.ajph.org). The additional effect of the VRA on Black deaths relative to White deaths was significant in the triple DID model using racialized group-stratified data (Table E, available as a supplement to the online version of this article at http://www.ajph.org).

The results of all of the robustness and sensitivity analyses were similar to the results of the main analysis in direction, magnitude, and significance (Tables F–I, available as a supplement to the online version of this article at http://www.ajph.org).

The exploratory analysis of long-term trends showed that there was an overall large decrease in infant mortality across VRA-exposure categories and racialized groups between the pre-VRA period of 1959 to 1965 and the post-VRA period of 2017 to 2021 (Table 1). The differential decrease among exposed compared with unexposed groups during this time period was not significant for the Black, White, or total population (Table J, available as a supplement to the online version of this article at http://www.ajph.org).

DISCUSSION

Our novel analyses provided evidence that, following passage of the VRA, Black infant deaths decreased more in covered counties than they did in noncovered counties. Between the pre-

TABLE 2— Difference-in-Differences Model Parameter Estimates for Models Fit in Former US Jim Crow States

	Post-VRA Period: 1966–1970, b (95% CI)	Post-VRA Period: 1971–1975, b (95% CI)	Post-VRA Period: 1976–1980, b (95% CI)
Total population			
Intercept	−22.9 (−73.2, 27.3)	−12.8 (−70.7, 45.2)	−9.2 (−80.5, 62.2)
Time period (post)	−28.8 (−40.4, −17.1)	−49.2 (−68.0, −30.4)	−65.5 (−89.9, −41.1)
Time period (post) × VRA (covered)	−13.1 (−29.3, 3.2)	−18.2 (−43.5, 7.1)	−19.9 (−51.0, 11.3)
Black infant deaths			
Intercept	5.3 (−8.3, 18.9)	13.9 (−5.3, 33.2)	18.1 (−13.4, 49.6)
Time period (post)	−8.9 (−14.1, −3.8)	−18.8 (−28.2, −9.4)	−26.6 (−40.3, −13.0)
Time period (post) × VRA (covered)	−11.4 (−21.0, −1.7)	−18.1 (−34.4, −1.9)	−21.6 (−42.4, −0.9)
White infant deaths			
Intercept	−13.0 (−25.7, −0.3)	−14.7 (−24.6, −4.9)	−16.9 (−29.9, −3.9)
Time period (post)	−21.0 (−27.2, −14.8)	−32.8 (−42.2, −23.5)	−42.6 (−53.7, −31.6)
Time period (post) × VRA (covered)	6.9 (−1.0, 14.7)	9.0 (−2.2, 20.2)	9.2 (−4.1, 22.6)

Note. CI = confidence interval; VRA = Voting Rights Act of 1965. Separate models were run for the total population and by racialized group, using data for a pre-VRA period (1959–1965) and for each of 3 post-VRA periods (1966–1970, 1971–1975, and 1976–1980). State fixed effects and baseline county characteristics are not displayed above. Please see Tables B through D (available as a supplement to the online version of this article at http://www.ajph.org) for the full regression output. Covered by VRA: AL, GA, LA, MS, SC, VA, 39 counties in NC, 9 counties in AZ. Not covered by VRA: AR, DE, DC, FL, KS, KY, MD, MO, NM, OK, TN, TX, WV, WY, 61 counties in NC, 5 counties in AZ.

VRA period of 1959 to 1965 and the post-VRA period of 1966 to 1970, this decrease amounted to over 6500 fewer Black infant deaths in covered counties, nearly 20% fewer deaths than would have been experienced in the absence of the VRA. Even so, despite the beneficial effect of the VRA, Black infant deaths remain higher than White infant deaths, controlling for population size, in all the post-VRA periods, up through 2021.

Limitations

A causal interpretation of our results relies on the assumptions of parallel trends and common shocks. One potential threat to the assumption of common shocks is the process of hospital desegregation that began in 1966. Although we included a variable in all regression models that indicated whether a county had at least 1 desegregated hospital, it is possible that some of the effect we detected could be due to differential effects of hospital desegregation in covered compared with noncovered counties. However, it is also possible that hospital desegregation is a mediator and on the causal pathway between the passage of the VRA and reductions in infant deaths because it occurred the year after the VRA passed. The assumption of common shocks is unlikely to hold through to the 2017–2021 post-VRA period, so the results of the exploratory analysis should be interpreted with caution.

A causal interpretation of our results also assumes that the composition of the underlying population does not change across the study period. We found that the Black population aged younger than 5 years may have decreased in covered counties but not in the noncovered counties. This could potentially confound the results of the DID regression. However, we included the population counts as a variable in our model, which should account for underlying population changes. Furthermore, we found evidence to support parallel trends in infant deaths in the pre-VRA period, which reduces concern of bias.

A limitation of this analysis relates to the accuracy of infant death records during the study period. It is possible that infant deaths are undercounted. However, investigations into the accuracy of vital statistic records from the 1940s to the 1960s indicate that by the early 1960s, nearly 100% of infant births and deaths were recorded. Furthermore, the official guidance from the National Center for Health Statistics is that the data files are usable, although they "have not been rigorously verified."[19] Some research has shown that infant deaths are more likely to be undercounted for Black infants and in rural and impoverished areas.[28,29] For our analysis, this could result in a disproportionate undercount of Black infant deaths in covered counties during the pre-VRA period (as covered counties overall have a higher percentage of Black residents, lower median income, and comparable population density), which would make our estimates conservative.

Results in Context

Guided by ecosocial theory, the additional reduction in Black infant mortality rates in VRA-covered counties can be understood as reflective of the changes the VRA produced to the embodied social, political, and economic conditions of Black Americans. The findings of this study are supported by and should be situated within the small bodies of work investigating (1) the effects of voter suppression and civic participation within public health and (2) the social and economic effects of the VRA.

Although no other studies have quantified the impact of the VRA on infant mortality, there is a body of work detailing how voting and civic participation is associated with improved public health. Several studies, all using post-1990 data, have demonstrated that there is an association between better health and voting—both that healthier people vote more and that voting is beneficial for health.[17,30] One study found that areas with high inequities in voter participation had lower self-rated health in 1990 to 1996.[31] Another study showed that individuals living in areas that had high barriers to voting (as defined by the Cost of Voting Index) had higher odds of being uninsured in 2017.[32]

Our findings that the VRA had a particularly beneficial effect on Black infant deaths in covered counties is in line with existing research on the social and economic effects of the VRA. Cascio and Washington investigated changes in state fund transfers to local county governments covered by the VRA compared with those that were not covered by the VRA. They found that VRA-covered counties with a high percentage of Black residents saw greater increases in state fund transfers from 1960 to 1980 than were seen in non-VRA comparison counties.[11] Aneja and Avenancio-Leon found larger decreases in the Black–White wage gap in VRA-covered counties from 1950 to 1980 compared with non-VRA-covered counties.[12] Facchini et al. found that the Black arrest rate decreased in VRA-covered counties compared with non-VRA counties from 1960 to 1981, whereas the White arrest rate did not change.[13] Increases in funding, increases in wages, and decreases in arrest rates all speak to improvements in the social and economic conditions, which are also known to improve health outcomes and are potential pathways explaining the results of this study. All these effects are factors that are known to be associated with health and health inequities.[14] Interestingly, Eubank and Fresh found differential increases in Black prison admission rates in covered compared with noncovered states from 1945 to 1980, which they attribute to backlash in response to Black political gains.[33] Investigating the role of backlash in response to Black enfranchisement and potential harms to public health and health equity warrants future research.

Public Health Implications

Our results add to the small but growing body of work analyzing the impact of political representation and political economy on population health. Although our study focuses on an historical 1965 policy change, the findings have contemporary relevance. First, individuals born prior to the VRA are still alive today (anyone born before 1965, or older than 58 years),[34] and assessing the health impacts of mass enfranchisement on their own health and potentially that of their children is important for understanding and addressing current health inequities. Second, our results highlight the need to investigate the health impacts of current attacks on voting rights, which are different in methods and scope to those used during the VRA time period, including restrictive voter ID laws, limitations to early and absentee voting, and gerrymandering,[15,16,30,32] because they plausibly could become embodied and affect population distributions of health and health inequities. AJPH

ABOUT THE AUTHORS

Tamara Rushovich and Nancy Krieger are with the Department of Social and Behavioral Sciences and Rachel C. Nethery is with the Department of Biostatistics, Harvard T. H. Chan School of Public Health, Boston, MA. Ariel White is with the Department of Political Science, Massachusetts Institute of Technology, Cambridge, MA.

CORRESPONDENCE

Correspondence should be sent to Tamara Rushovich, MPH, PhD Candidate, Department of Social and Behavioral Sciences, Harvard T. H. Chan School of Public Health, 677 Huntington Ave, Boston, MA 02115 (e-mail: trushovich@g.harvard.edu). Reprints can be ordered at http://www.ajph.org by clicking the "Reprints" link.

PUBLICATION INFORMATION

Full Citation: Rushovich T, Nethery RC, White A, Krieger N. 1965 US Voting Rights Act impact on Black and Black versus White infant death rates in Jim Crow states, 1959–1980 and 2017–2021. *Am J Public Health*. 2024;114(3):300–308.

Acceptance Date: October 24, 2023.

DOI: https://doi.org/10.2105/AJPH.2023.307518

ORCID iDs:

Tamara Rushovich https://orcid.org/0000-0001-5344-0067

CONTRIBUTORS

T. Rushovich initiated the study and led writing of the manuscript, conceptualizing the study design, acquiring the data, conducting the analyses, and interpreting the results. T. Rushovich, A. White, and N. Krieger contributed to conceptualizing the study, designing the analyses, interpreting the results, and preparing the manuscript. All authors approved the final version for submission.

ACKNOWLEDGMENTS

We acknowledge and thank Jarvis Chen, PhD, and Soroush Moallef for their assistance with acquiring and utilizing the 2017–2021 NCHS mortality data (written permission: October 24, 2023).

CONFLICTS OF INTEREST

No authors have any conflicts of interest to declare.

HUMAN PARTICIPANT PROTECTION

This study was reviewed by the Harvard T. H. Chan institutional review board (IRB21-1615), was determined not to be human participant research, and was deemed exempt.

REFERENCES

1. Oyez. Shelby County v Holder. Available at: https://www.oyez.org/cases/2012/12-96. Accessed October 28, 2021.
2. Dawes DE. *The Political Determinants of Health.* Baltimore, MD: Johns Hopkins Press; 2020.
3. Krieger N, Testa C, Chen JT, Hanage WP, McGregor AJ. Relationship of political ideology of US federal and state elected officials and key covid pandemic outcomes following vaccine rollout to adults: April 2021–March 2022. *Lancet Reg Health Am.* 2022;16:100384. https://doi.org/10.1016/j.lana.2022.100384
4. Krieger N, Boyd RW, De Maio F, Maybank A. Medicine's privileged gatekeepers: producing harmful ignorance about racism and health. *Health Affairs Blog.* May 9, 2021. https://doi.org/10.1377/forefront.20210415.305480
5. American Civil Liberties Union. Voting Rights Act: major dates in history. Available at: https://www.aclu.org/voting-rights-act-major-dates-history. Accessed December 23, 2022.
6. Murray P. *States' Laws on Race and Color.* Athens: University of Georgia Press; 1997.
7. US Dept of Justice. Section 4 of The Voting Rights Act. May 5, 2020. Available at: https://www.justice.gov/crt/section-4-voting-rights-act. Accessed December 23, 2022.
8. Grofman B, Handley L. The impact of the Voting Rights Act on Black representation in Southern state legislatures. *Legis Stud Q.* 1991;16(1):111–128. https://doi.org/10.2307/439970
9. Husted TA, Kenny LW. The effect of the expansion of the voting franchise on the size of government. *J Polit Econ.* 1997;105(1):54–82.
10. Schuit S, Rogowski JC. Race, representation, and the Voting Rights Act. *Am J Pol Sci.* 2017;61:513–526. https://doi.org/10.1111/ajps.12284
11. Cascio EU, Washington E. Valuing the vote: the redistribution of voting rights and state funds following the Voting Rights Act of 1965. *Q J Econ.* 2014;129(1):379–433. https://doi.org/10.1093/qje/qjt028
12. Aneja A, Avenancio-Leon CF. The effect of political power on labor market inequality: evidence from the 1965 Voting Rights Act. October 2020. Available at: https://equitablegrowth.org/working-papers/the-effect-of-political-power-on-labor-market-inequality-evidence-from-the-1965-voting-rights-act. Accessed August 9, 2021.
13. Facchini G, Knight BG, Testa C. The franchise, policing, and race: evidence from arrests data and the Voting Rights Act. National Bureau of Economic Research; 2020. https://doi.org/10.3386/w27463
14. Berkman L, Kawachi I, Glymour MM, eds. *Social Epidemiology.* 2nd ed. New York, NY: Oxford University Press; 2014.
15. Hing AK. The right to vote, the right to health: voter suppression as a determinant of racial health disparities. *J Health Dispar Res Pract.* 2019;12(6):48–62.
16. Homan PA, Brown TH. Sick and tired of being excluded: structural racism in disenfranchisement as a threat to population health equity. *Health Aff.* 2022;41(2):219–227. https://doi.org/10.1377/hlthaff.2021.01414
17. Kim S, Kim CY, You MS. Civic participation and self-rated health: a cross-national multi-level analysis using the World Value Survey. *J Prev Med Public Health.* 2015;48(1):18–27. https://doi.org/10.3961/jpmph.14.031
18. Krieger N. *Epidemiology and the People's Health: Theory and Context.* Oxford University Press; 2011.
19. National Bureau of Economic Research. Mortality data—vital statistics NCHS multiple cause of death data. Available at: https://www.nber.org/research/data/mortality-data-vital-statistics-nchs-multiple-cause-death-data. Accessed December 15, 2022.
20. Ruggles S, Flood S, Goeken R, et al. IPUMS National Historical Geographic Information System: Version 17.0 (1940, 1950, 1960, 1970, 1980 Census). 2020. https://doi.org/10.18128/D010.V10.0
21. Haines MR, Inter-University Consortium for Political and Social Research. Historical, demographic, economic, and social data: The United States, 1790–2002. May 21, 2010. https://doi.org/10.3886/ICPSR02896.v3
22. National Center for Health Statistics. Deaths (mortality)—multiple cause of death, states, and all counties—detailed (2017–2021), as compiled from data provided by the 57 vital statistics jurisdictions through the Vital Statistics Cooperative Program. Available at: https://www.cdc.gov/nchs/nvss/nvss-restricted-data.htm. Accessed July 2023.
23. Gortmaker SL, Wise PH. The first injustice: socioeconomic disparities, health services technology, and infant mortality. *Annu Rev Sociol.* 1997;23:147–170.
24. Centers for Disease Control and Prevention. Infant mortality. June 22, 2022. Available at: https://www.cdc.gov/reproductivehealth/maternalinfanthealth/infantmortality.htm. Accessed November 15, 2022.
25. Reidpath DD, Allotey P. Infant mortality rate as an indicator of population health. *J Epidemiol Community Health.* 2003;57(5):344–346. https://doi.org/10.1136/jech.57.5.344
26. Krieger N, Waterman PD, Spasojevic J, Li W, Maduro G, Van Wye G. Public health monitoring of privilege and deprivation with the Index of Concentration at the Extremes. *Am J Public Health.* 2016;106(2):256–263. https://doi.org/10.2105/AJPH.2015.302955
27. Feng C. Zero-inflated models for adjusting varying exposures: a cautionary note on the pitfalls of using offset. *J Appl Stat.* 49(1):1–23. https://doi.org/10.1080/02664763.2020.1796943
28. Rogers PB, Council CR, Abernathy JR. Testing death registration completeness in a group of premature infants. *Public Health Rep (1896).* 1961;76(8):717–726.
29. McCarthy BJ, Terry J, Rochat RW, Tyler CW. The underregistration of neonatal deaths: Georgia 1974–77. *Am J Public Health.* 1980;70(9):977–982. https://doi.org/10.2105/AJPH.70.9.977
30. Brown CL, Raza D, Pinto AD. Voting, health and interventions in healthcare settings: a scoping review. *Public Health Rev.* 2020;41(1):16. https://doi.org/10.1186/s40985-020-00133-6
31. Blakely TA, Kennedy BP, Kawachi I. Socioeconomic inequality in voting participation and self-rated health. *Am J Public Health.* 2001;91(1):99–104. https://doi.org/10.2105/ajph.91.1.99
32. Pabayo R, Liu SY, Grinshteyn E, Cook DM, Muennig P. Barriers to voting and access to health insurance among US adults: a cross-sectional study. *Lancet Reg Health Am.* 2021;2:100026. https://doi.org/10.1016/j.lana.2021.100026
33. Eubank N, Fresh A. Enfranchisement and incarceration after the 1965 Voting Rights Act. *Am Polit Sci Rev.* 2022;116(3):791–806. https://doi.org/10.1017/S0003055421001337
34. Krieger N, Chen JT, Coull B, Waterman PD, Beckfield J. The unique impact of abolition of Jim Crow laws on reducing inequities in infant death rates and implications for choice of comparison groups in analyzing societal determinants of health. *Am J Public Health.* 2013;103(12):2234–2244. https://doi.org/10.2105/AJPH.2013.301350

Airborne Lead Exposure and Childhood Cognition: The Environmental Influences on Child Health Outcomes (ECHO) Cohort (2003–2022)

Lisa M. Gatzke-Kopp, PhD, Michael Willoughby, PhD, Amii M. Kress, PhD, Kristen McArthur, ScM, Cara Wychgram, MPP, David C. Folch, PhD, Steve Brunswasser, PhD, Dana Dabelea, MD, PhD, Amy J. Elliott, PhD, Tina Hartert, MD, MPH, Margaret Karagas, PhD, Cindy T. McEvoy, MD, MCR, James A. VanDerslice, PhD, Robert O. Wright, MD, MPH, and Rosalind J. Wright, MD; on Behalf of Program Collaborators for Environmental Influences on Child Health Outcomes

Objectives. To examine whether a previously reported association between airborne lead exposure and children's cognitive function replicates across a geographically diverse sample of the United States.

Methods. Residential addresses of children (< 5 years) were spatially joined to the Risk-Screening Environmental Indicators model of relative airborne lead toxicity. Cognitive outcomes for children younger than 8 years were available for 1629 children with IQ data and 1476 with measures of executive function (EF; inhibitory control, cognitive flexibility). We used generalized linear models using generalized estimating equations to examine the associations of lead, scaled by interquartile range (IQR), accounting for individual- and area-level confounders.

Results. An IQR increase in airborne lead was associated with a 0.74-point lower mean IQ score ($b = -0.74$; 95% confidence interval = −1.00, −0.48). The association between lead and EF was nonlinear and was modeled with a knot at the 97.5th percentile of lead in our sample. Lead was significantly associated with lower mean inhibitory control but not with cognitive flexibility. This effect was stronger among males for both IQ and inhibitory control.

Conclusions. Early-life exposure to airborne lead is associated with lower cognitive functioning. (*Am J Public Health*. 2024;114(3):309–318. https://doi.org/10.2105/AJPH.2023.307519)

AJPH March 2024, Vol. 114, No. 3

The neurotoxic effects of lead on children's intellectual and cognitive development are well known.[1] Although lead is cleared from the blood in the course of approximately 1 month, the bioaccumulating properties of lead give it a half-life of 2 to 3 years in neural tissue.[2] Evidence suggests that males may be more sensitive to the neurotoxic effects of lead, although more epidemiological research in human samples is needed.[3]

Despite a dramatic decrease in children's blood lead levels in recent decades,[4,5] significant disparities in lead exposure persist. Particularly high risk of exposure occurs in regions with older and poorly kept housing, or in regions where poor municipal management of water systems has allowed for contamination from corroded pipes.[6,7] However, less research has examined the effects of airborne exposure associated with industrial emissions.

Atmospheric lead levels have fluctuated across the globe and throughout history as a function of regional changes in pollution production (e.g., smelting, manufacturing) and environmental policies (e.g., removal of lead from gasoline).[5] Individuals can be exposed to airborne lead directly through inhalation, or through ingestion or absorption as airborne lead settles into soil or contaminates ground water.[2] In the United States, airborne pollution is monitored by the Environmental Protection Agency (EPA), which models exposure for sources of emission in the Toxic Release Inventory, accounting for dynamic meteorological factors that affect the range of dispersion at a resolution of half-square-mile (810-m) cells. The publicly available Risk-Screening Environmental Indicators (RSEI) database provides quantified estimates of relative toxicity potential of chemicals from the Toxic Release Inventory, accounting for the route of exposure (e.g., inhalation) and the impact of sustained exposure on human health. Using these data, we previously examined how area-level airborne lead toxicity risk in a child's first 3 years of life related to cognitive function in the preschool period in a sample of 849 children living in nonmetropolitan mid-Atlantic regions.[8] Results revealed an association between higher airborne lead toxicity risk and lower estimated IQ at age 3 years, as well as lower performance on executive function (EF) tasks at ages 3, 4, and 5 years, suggesting that the effects of this exposure are persistent. These findings are consistent with mounting evidence that no degree of lead exposure can be presumed to be innocuous.[9] In the present study, we sought to replicate our previous findings using the Environmental Influences on Child Health Outcomes (ECHO) Cohort. This consortium incorporates greater geographic and socioeconomic diversity, allowing for a replication that is more broadly representative of the United States.

METHODS

The ECHO Cohort combines 69 ongoing pregnancy and pediatric cohort sites across the United States into a single cohort with the goal of studying environmental factors associated with child health.[10] Cohort sites were eligible for the current analysis if 30 or more children had high-quality geocoded residential address data (i.e., address matched to a point address feature or a specific street address) between birth and age 3 years, and at least 1 measure of cognitive function before age 8 years. Descriptions of included cohort sites are presented in Table A (available as a supplement to the online version of this article at http://www.ajph.org). We excluded children born after 2017 from the current analysis, allowing all included participants to have at least 3 years of exposure data, as at the time of analysis RSEI data were available through calendar year 2020. We excluded participants from the cohort sites included in the first study to evaluate RSEI lead and cognition[8] and those with a diagnosis of autism spectrum disorder (n = 95; Figure A, available as a supplement to the online version of this article at http://www.ajph.org).

Of the 60 553 ECHO Cohort participants available as of March 2022, 13 cohort sites (4364 children) administered IQ measures and 30 cohort sites (1948 children) administered relevant EF measures; 1629 children from 6 cohort sites and 1334 children from 10 cohort sites met inclusion criteria for the full-scale IQ and EF samples, respectively. Within the EF sample, we evaluated 1241 children for inhibitory control (measured with Flanker Task) and 1298 for cognitive flexibility (measured with Dimensional Change Card Sort [DCCS]). Most (89.4%) of those included had both EF measures. Sample characteristics for the ECHO Cohort and the 2 subsamples (i.e., IQ and EF) are reported in Table 1. We conducted analyses separately for the 3 cognitive outcomes (i.e., IQ, Flanker, DCCS).

Figure 1 illustrates the relative toxicity estimates of airborne lead aggregated to county in the United States using the most recently available (2020) RSEI values. Counties with participants included in the analyses are noted with symbols at the county centroid (participants in IQ, EF, or both samples). Participants in the IQ sample resided in 237 counties across 41 states, and participants in the EF sample resided in 188 counties across 36 states. Included children were born between 2003 and 2017, with the majority (66.3%–76.2%) born between 2010 and 2014. Only children in the IQ sample had birth years prior to 2010 (20.6%).

Measures

Lead exposure. To account for residential moves, we created a monthly address history file for each child. In instances where data were unclear about the precise timing of residential moves, we used adjacent known addresses to fill the months from the midpoint of the identified gap. We geocoded addresses in ArcGIS Pro Streetmap Premium Geocoder (Esri, Redlands, CA) to generate a precise latitude and longitude for integration with the lead exposure data. We used only addresses that could be mapped to a point (> 85% of addresses). Low-precision (excluded) addresses were not systematically associated with child birth year, age at outcome assessment, or geographic region. Lead exposure

TABLE 1— Sociodemographic, Birth, and Area-Level Characteristics for the Environmental Influences on Child Health Outcomes (ECHO) Cohort, Full-Scale IQ, and Executive Functioning Samples: United States, 2003–2017

	No. (%), Mean ±SD, or Mean ±SD (IQR)		
	ECHO Cohort (n = 60 553 Children and 69 Cohorts)	Full-Scale IQ[a] (n = 1629 Children and 6 Cohorts)	Executive Functioning[a] (n = 1343 Children and 10 Cohorts)
Child characteristics			
Child's sex			
Male	30 934 (51.7)	836 (51.3)	685 (51.0)
Female	28 925 (48.3)	793 (48.7)	658 (49.0)
Child's race			
White	34 136 (62.9)	1 010 (64.1)	837 (63.5)
Black	8 553 (15.8)	125 (7.9)	136 (10.3)
Multiple	5 941 (10.9)	270 (17.2)	154 (11.7)
All others	5 670 (10.4)	170 (10.8)	192 (14.6)
Child's ethnicity			
Non-Hispanic	41 194 (71.9)	1 329 (82.2)	988 (73.6)
Hispanic	16 891 (27.9)	287 (17.8)	354 (26.4)
Birth year			
Before 2010	22 505 (37.2)	335 (20.6)	0 (0.0)
2010–2014	16 891 (27.9)	1 182 (72.6)	890 (66.3)
2015 and later	21 157 (34.9)	112 (6.9)	453 (33.7)
Preterm (< 37 wk gestation)			
No	46 760 (85.5)	1 331 (83.1)	1 032 (77.0)
Yes	7 915 (14.5)	270 (16.9)	309 (23.0)
Low birth weight (< 2500 g)			
No	38 484 (86.9)	1 338 (85.5)	1 031 (78.0)
Yes	5 777 (13.1)	226 (14.5)	290 (22.0)
Mean age at assessment, y	. . .	5.9 ± 0.8	5.0 ± 1.0
Birthing parent characteristics			
Age at delivery, y	29.8 ± 5.9	30.8 ± 5.6	30.3 ± 5.7
Education			
< High school	4 932 (9.4)	106 (6.8)	58 (4.3)
High school/GED	9 014 (17.2)	183 (11.8)	126 (9.4)
Some college or more	38 486 (73.4)	1 263 (81.4)	1 152 (86.2)
Tobacco during pregnancy			
No	41 081 (89.5)	1 143 (92.8)	1 188 (89.8)
Yes	4 802 (10.5)	78 (7.2)	135 (10.2)
Area-level characteristics[b]			
RSEI lead toxicity score	. . .	2.1 ± 2.8 (2.3)	1.2 ± 1.7 (1.5)
SVI socioeconomic status (SES) theme tertiles			
Low vulnerability (< 0.34)	. . .	867 (53.2)	637 (47.4)
Moderate vulnerability (0.34–0.64)	. . .	440 (27.0)	407 (30.3)
High vulnerability (> 0.66)	. . .	322 (19.8)	299 (22.3)
SVI SES theme (mean [SD])	. . .	0.4 ± 0.3	0.4 ± 0.3

Continued

TABLE 1— Continued

	No. (%), Mean ±SD, or Mean ±SD (IQR)		
	ECHO Cohort (n = 60 553 Children and 69 Cohorts)	Full-Scale IQ[a] (n = 1629 Children and 6 Cohorts)	Executive Functioning[a] (n = 1343 Children and 10 Cohorts)
Rural–urban commuting area (RUCA)			
Urban	. . .	1 158 (71.1)	1 293 (96.3)
Rural	. . .	471 (28.9)	50 (3.7)
Census tract–level % pre-1980s housing			
Low (≤ 46.07%)	. . .	255 (15.7)	463 (34.5)
Moderate (46.08%–74.64%)	. . .	695 (42.7)	426 (31.7)
High (≥ 74.65)	. . .	679 (41.7)	454 (33.8)
Housing age (% of census tract before 1980)	. . .	66.8 ± 21.2	55.9 ± 29.0
Census region			
Midwest	. . .	141 ± 8.7	208 ± 15.5
Northeast	. . .	1 164 ± 71.5	167 ± 12.4
South	. . .	35 ± 2.2	196 ± 14.6
West	. . .	289 ± 17.7	772 ± 57.5

Note. IQR = interquartile range; SVI = Social Vulnerability Index.
[a]A total of 183 participants were in both IQ and executive functioning samples.
[b]Area-level characteristics are not presented for the full ECHO sample as addresses are not available for the full ECHO-wide cohort. Lead exposure is quantified from the Risk-Screening Environmental Indicators (RSEI) Model lead toxicity score (ToxConc). Percentage of census tracts with pre-1980 housing is drawn from the American Community Survey (ACS) 5-year estimates. ACS data from 2009, 2014, and 2019 were applied to address history data from 2002 to 2009, 2010 to 2014, and 2015 to 2019, respectively.

was based on the EPA's RSEI Model microdata (version 2.3.10) 2003 through 2020.[11] The RSEI microdata provide a unitless index of relative concentration in an 810 × 810 m (1/2 × 1/2 mile) grid as a function of the substance's toxicity when inhaled. We quantified total exposure as the average monthly RSEI value up to outcome ascertainment (for outcomes measured before age 5 years) or month 60 (i.e., age 5 years, for outcomes measured after this age). We winsorized extreme RSEI values at the 1st and 99th percentiles. For analyses, we modeled RSEI lead data as a continuous untransformed measure and also scaled them by the interquartile range (IQR) for interpretability. Table 1 reports the RSEI values for each sample. Sample average relative toxicity scores were higher than the 2020 average for the United States (0.79). Participant scores ranged from 0 to 18.3 in the IQ sample and from 0 to 12.0 in the EF sample.

Cognitive outcomes. ECHO cohorts varied with regard to the nature and timing of cognitive assessments. Among cohorts that measured IQ, assessment ages ranged from 4 to 7.9 years (median = 6; IQR = 5.3–6.4). Among cohorts that measured EF, assessment ages ranged from 3 to 7.9 years (median = 5.3; IQR = 4.6–6.0). For participants with multiple assessments, we selected the assessment closest to age 5 years.

We assessed full-scale IQ with the appropriate Wechsler Scale[12] (i.e., *Wechsler Preschool and Primary Scale of Intelligence*, 3rd or 4th editions, and *Wechsler Abbreviated Scale of Intelligence*, 2nd–5th editions) and harmonized it for use in the IQ analyses. We collected most of the IQ data using cohort-specific protocols prior to the implementation of the ECHO-wide data collection protocol. Harmonization of these data varied by cohort (e.g., averaging of available subtests). Mean sample IQ score was 102 (SD = 14.6) and ranged from 42 to 149. IQ data for these analyses were collected between 2011 and 2022.

We examined 2 age-appropriate subtests from the NIH Toolbox as indicators of EF. We used the Flanker Task as a measure of inhibitory control based on the age-corrected standard score for this task that was generated by test developers.[13] Scores ranged from 54 to 135 (mean = 100; SD = 13.4). We used the DCCS as a

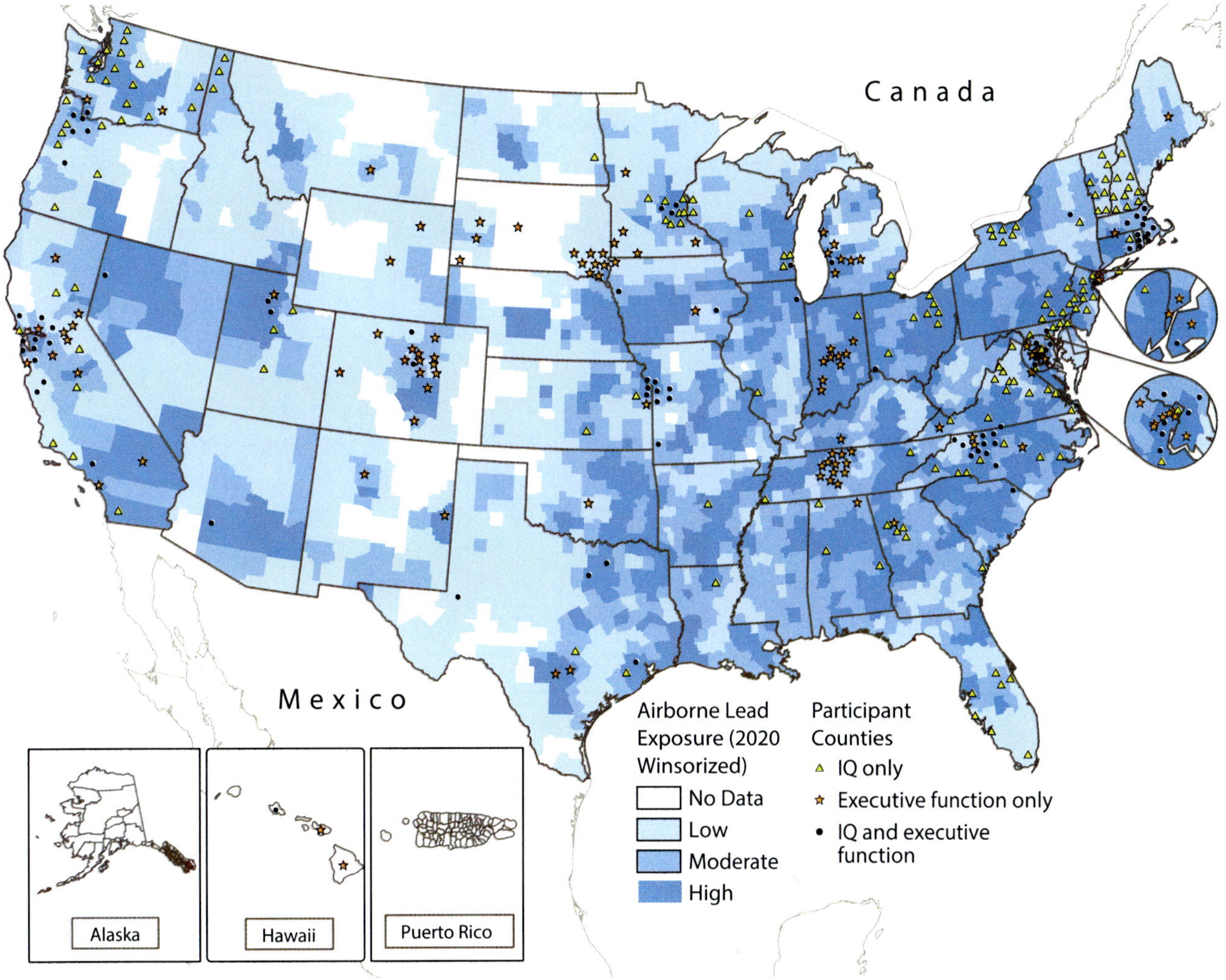

FIGURE 1— Study Participants and County-Level Risk-Screening Environmental Indicators (RSEI) Lead Toxicity Scores: United States, 2020

Note. RSEI lead toxicity scores are illustrated by county using the 2020 RSEI Model lead toxicity scores with extreme values (defined as 1st and 99th percentile) winsorized. Scores may not correspond to exposure values at the time of the participants' birth. Symbols represent county centroids where participants resided and which cognitive outcome data they contributed.

measure of cognitive flexibility, and also computed it as an age-corrected standard score following test developer guidelines.[14] Scores ranged from 54 to 145 (mean = 98; SD = 13.9). EF outcome data were collected between 2016 and 2022.

Confounders. We identified potential confounders a priori at the individual and census tract levels based on theory, previous studies, and data availability. Descriptive values are reported in Table 1, and correlations are reported in Table B (available as a supplement to the online version of this article at http://www.ajph.org).

We adjusted for characteristics of the child, including sex assigned at birth, age at cognitive assessment (continuous, centered at 5 years; IQ sample only), and preterm status (< 37 weeks vs ≥ 37 weeks gestation). We also adjusted for characteristics of the birthing parent with a theoretical impact on the individual child, including age at delivery (continuous, centered at 30 years), educational attainment (< high school, high school, or > high school), and prenatal smoking (ever vs never).

We used geocoded addresses joined to census tract–level data to characterize indicators of neighborhood-level socioeconomic status (SES), urbanicity, and potential for lead exposure via older homes.

The Social Vulnerability Index (SVI), developed by the Centers for Disease Control and Prevention's Agency for Toxic Substances and Disease Registry, describes the relative vulnerability of every US census tract based on 15 social factors that are grouped into 4 themes. The present analyses utilized the SES theme, which reflects income, education, and employment data. Lower SVI values reflect less social vulnerability (i.e., higher SES). For analyses, we categorized SVI values as tertiles (high SES [reference] ≤ 0.33; medium SES = 0.34–0.66; low SES ≥ 0.66).

We used rural–urban commuting area (RUCA) codes,[15] developed by the Department of Agriculture's Economic Research Service, to identify metropolitan versus nonmetropolitan census tracts. The RUCA values are based on measures of population density, urbanization, and daily commuting and range from 1 (metropolitan) to 10 (rural). We used the closest corresponding RUCA values (from 2000 or 2010) to classify each residential address entry. We used the most current (v. 1.1) thresholds provided by the Rural Health Research Center to classify participants as residing in metropolitan or nonmetropolitan areas.

To control for potential lead exposure in the home, we used the 2009, 2014, and 2019[16] American Community Survey (ACS) 5-year estimates to calculate the census tract–level proportion of pre-1980s housing because units built prior to 1978 typically contain lead-based paint. We applied 2009 ACS data to 2003–2009 participant residential history records, 2014 data to 2010–2014 records, and 2019 data to 2015–2022 records. The percentage of housing units within tracts with units built before 1980 was parameterized as tertiles based on national distribution in 2019 ACS for analyses (low [reference] ≤ 46.07%; moderate = 46.08%–74.64%; high 3: ≥ 74.65%).

Statistical Analyses

We conducted analyses using Stata version 17.0 (StataCorp LP, College Station, TX) and R version 4.2.2.

For the relatively small proportion of missing covariate data, we assumed data were missing at random and used the multiple imputation by chained equation (MICE) method[17] (10 imputations with 10 iterations each) for IQ (< 5% maternal education, preterm, low birth weight, maternal age; 24% prenatal tobacco use) and EF (< 5% maternal education, preterm, low birth weight, maternal age, prenatal tobacco use) study populations separately. We imputed missing confounder data with indicators for original cohort and cohort design (i.e., enriched for preterm births and neonatal intensive care unit) admission at birth or general population), birth characteristics (e.g., neonatal intensive care unit admission, gestational age, birth weight), family socioeconomic characteristics (e.g., income, birthing parent's marital status). We calculated all regression estimates using the average of the 10 estimates derived from the imputed data sets, and we estimated standard errors of the parameters using Rubin's rules (Table D, available as a supplement to the online version of this article at http://www.ajph.org).

We also estimated the intraclass correlation coefficient (ICC) to examine potential clustering of participants by cohort site (i.e., the original study that recruited the participant) and census tract. Cohort site ICCs were 0.17 for IQ, 0.07 for Flanker, and 0.06 for DCCS. Given the ICC value of greater than 0.10 observed for the IQ sample, we used generalized linear models using generalized estimating equations (exchangeable correlation structure and robust variance estimates) to examine the associations of RSEI lead measures while accounting for within-cohort site clustering.

We examined the functional form of the relationship between RSEI lead exposure and cognitive outcomes. On the basis of an examination of scatterplots and LOWESS curves, we observed a nonlinear relationship between lead and EF outcomes. We then compared quasi-likelihood under independence model criteria (QIC) for nested models containing (1) linear parameterization of lead only, (2) quadratic parameterization, and (3) spline with knot at the 97.5th percentile of lead exposure. For both EF outcomes, models containing a spline with knot at the 97.5th percentile of lead yielded a lower QIC; lead was therefore parameterized by 2 terms with a knot at the 97.5th percentile of lead for the EF models. Our focus was on the main lead parameter (i.e., describing those in the bottom 97.5% of lead exposure), as the top tail of lead exposure comprised fewer than 35 children.

For all outcomes, we started with unadjusted models of the association between RSEI lead and cognition. We then adjusted for individual-level confounders, including birthing parent's age at delivery, educational attainment, and prenatal smoking; child's sex assigned at birth; age at outcome assessment (IQ sample only); and preterm status. Finally, we added area-level confounders: SES (SVI), urbanicity (RUCA), and proportion of housing stock built before 1980.

Sensitivity Analyses

We conducted 3 sensitivity analyses to examine the robustness of the results. First, we omitted individuals whose cognitive function scores were more than 3 standard deviations beyond the norm. Second, we considered the impacts of area-level confounders sequentially to determine whether any specific covariate was unduly influential in the model. Third, we conducted a "leave-one-out analysis" to determine whether any specific cohort site exerted undue influence on results.

Moderation by Sex

Given evidence that lead exposure may have sexually dimorphic effects, we estimated sex-specific models, and modeled a lead-by-sex interaction to examine whether child's sex at birth moderated the association between potential lead exposure and cognitive outcomes. We considered a 2-sided *P* value less than .10 for the interaction term as evidence of effect modification.

RESULTS

Bivariate correlations between RSEI lead values, continuous confounders, and cognitive outcomes are provided in online Tables B and C. Individual differences in children's IQ were not correlated with RSEI lead exposure ($r = 0.04$, not significant), but were correlated with SVI, pre-1980 housing, birthing parent's age, and child's gestational age ($r = -0.32$–0.28; $P < .05$). Children's EF was greater among those residing in regions of higher SES and who were born closer to term. Only inhibitory control (but not cognitive flexibility) was associated with the regional proportion of pre-1980s housing stock. Both inhibitory control and cognitive flexibility showed a significant negative association between RSEI lead exposure for the bottom 97.5% of the sample ($r = -0.13$ and -0.06, respectively; $P < .05$). Bivariate associations were only considered for continuous measures.

The fully adjusted associations between the average amount of early-life potential airborne lead exposure (i.e., up to outcome or age 5 years) and children's cognitive outcomes (mean IQ = 5.9; mean EF = 5.0) are summarized in Table 2. Individual differences in RSEI lead exposure were significantly inversely associated with IQ (b = −0.31; 95% confidence interval [95% CI] = −0.41, −0.20). An IQR increase in airborne lead was associated with a 0.74-point lower mean IQ score (95% CI = −1.00, −0.48).

TABLE 2— Adjusted Associations Between Risk-Screening Environmental Indicators (RSEI) Lead and Cognition in the Environmental Influences on Child Health Outcomes (ECHO) Cohort for the Full Sample and Sex-Stratified Analyses: United States, 2003–2017

		Executive Function[a]	
	Full-Scale IQ, No. or b (95% CI)	Inhibitory Control (Flanker), No. or b (95% CI)	Cognitive Flexibility (DCCS), No. or b (95% CI)
Total sample	1629	1241	1298
Per unit Δ airborne lead	−0.31 (−0.41, −0.20)	−0.67 (−1.25, −0.08)	−0.09 (−0.55, 0.37)
Per IQR Δ airborne lead	−0.74 (−1.00, −0.48)	−1.13 (−2.13, −0.14)	−0.15 (−0.93, 0.62)
Sex-stratified models[b]			
Male participants	836	635	657
Per unit Δ airborne lead	−0.60 (−0.81, −0.38)	−0.93 (−1.76, −0.11)	−0.12 (−0.80, 0.56)
Per IQR Δ airborne lead	−1.46 (−1.99, −0.92)	−1.58 (−2.98, −0.19)	−0.20 (−1.54, 0.99)
Female participants	793	606	641
Per unit Δ airborne lead	0.13 (−0.05, 0.31)	−0.42 (−0.85, 0.01)	0.08 (−0.28, 0.43)
Per IQR Δ airborne lead	0.32 (−0.12, 0.76)	−0.71 (−1.43, 0.02)	0.13 (−0.47, 0.73)

Note. CI = confidence interval; DCCS = Dimensional Card Change Sort. All models were fully adjusted for child's sex, age at assessment (IQ only), preterm birth (yes/no), maternal age at delivery, maternal education, prenatal smoking, social vulnerability index, rural-urban commuting area code, and census-block age of housing stock. Age was not included in executive function outcome models because NIH Toolbox scores are age adjusted.

[a]Following evidence of nonlinearity in the executive function models, a spline term was applied with a knot at 97.5th percentile of RSEI lead values in our sample. For executive function models, lead is modeled as $b_{(\leq 97.\text{fifth percentile})}$. Results for b (spline) = $b_{(> 97.\text{fifth percentile})}$ are presented in Table F (available as a supplement to the online version of this article at http://www.ajph.org).

[b]An additional fully adjusted model including a sex × lead interaction suggested moderation by sex (results not presented). Moderation was significant for the IQ model (*P* = .002) and inhibitory control (*P* = .084), but not for cognitive flexibility.

RSEI lead exposure was also associated with worse performance on the inhibitory control task for children in the bottom 97.5% of lead exposure (b = −0.67; 95% CI = −1.25, −0.08). An IQR increase in lead was associated with a 1.13-unit lower inhibitory control task score (95% CI = -2.13, −0.14). Although not statistically significant, a similar pattern of results emerged for the cognitive flexibility task (b = −0.09; 95% CI -0.55, 0.37). Children with the highest lead exposure (i.e., above the knot at 97.5th percentile of lead) did not follow this pattern, although these findings should be interpreted with caution given the small sample size. Model results for the complete spline model are presented in Table F (available as a supplement to the online version of this article at http://www.ajph.org), and plots of fitted values with 95% confidence intervals are presented in online Figure B.

We conducted a series of sensitivity tests to inform the robustness of these results. No extreme outliers were observed for EF scores, but a small number of IQ scores (n < 5) exceeded 3 standard deviations beyond the mean. The exclusion of these participants had only a modest impact on the effect estimate (b = −0.28; 95% CI = −0.39, −0.18) and no influence on substantive interpretation. We conducted a series of analyses with models that included the full set of individual-level confounders and that introduced the area-level confounders (SVI, RUCA, pre-1980 housing stock) one at a time. In general, the consideration of each area-level confounder resulted in negligible attenuation to point estimates from the fully adjusted model (summarized in Table E (available as a supplement to the online version of this article at http://www.ajph.org).

To ensure that effects were not specific to any cohort site, we reestimated the fully adjusted models leaving 1 cohort site out at a time. Forest plots of point estimates are presented in online Figures C and D. The consistency of estimates across models supports the robustness of this association.

Finally, we examined whether child's sex moderated the observed associations. The sex × lead interaction term was significant for the IQ model (*P* = .002). Results of the fully adjusted IQ model stratified by sex are reported in Table 2. For the IQ model, associations were significant only for males (b = −0.60; 95% CI = −0.81, −0.38). To examine the magnitude of this effect, we computed the model implied value of IQ for males whose airborne lead exposure was at the 10th percentile (101.9) versus that of males whose exposure was at the 90th percentile (99.3), which corresponds to an effect of approximately 2.6 IQ points.

The sex × lead interaction term did not reach significance for the model of cognitive flexibility (DCCS; *P* = .78) but was significant for the model of inhibitory control (Flanker; *P* = .08). In stratified analyses, effects were significant only for males (b = −0.93; 95% CI = −1.76, −0.11), with a weaker effect observed in females (b = −0.42; 95% CI = −0.85, 0.01).

DISCUSSION

Despite efforts to reduce environmental sources of lead exposure, airborne exposure varies appreciably across the United States. Using data pooled across 14 cohorts of children geographically dispersed across the United States, we found an association between greater relative magnitude of airborne lead exposure and lower IQ and EF in children aged 3 to 7 years, an effect that was not driven by any specific cohort site. Coupled with previous evidence of this association in nonmetropolitan areas,[8] our findings indicate a modest but significant effect of airborne lead exposure on children's cognitive development. Notably, males were more sensitive to the detrimental effects of airborne lead.

Significant associations were observed for both IQ and inhibitory control, consistent with previous evidence that blood lead levels correlate with a range of cognitive and academic metrics.[5] Associations between airborne lead and IQ were linear, whereas the association with EF was not. Nonlinear associations have been reported across a variety of previous studies, with evidence that the largest relative impact occurs in the lower exposure brackets.[5] A previous pooled analysis estimated a 6.2-point decline in IQ per increase in blood lead (up to 10 μg/dL), with the proportional magnitude of impact on IQ declining at higher values.[18] Contrary to a threshold effect in which a certain dosage must be reached before symptoms emerge, this pattern suggests that mechanisms underlying cognitive impairment are rapidly saturated.[5] However, the nonlinear effect observed in the present data suggests a reversal of association at airborne lead exposure exceeding the 97.5th percentile. Such an effect is inconsistent with the known neurotoxic effects of lead exposure, and caution is warranted in interpreting this effect given the very small number of participants with exposure values in that range. It is possible that this effect reflects a selection bias with regard to who, among individuals residing in high-exposure regions, elects to participate in research.

Previous work has suggested that males are more vulnerable to the effects of adverse conditions during neurodevelopment generally,[19] and specifically with regard to the neurodevelopmental effects of lead exposure.[3] These findings, along with evidence that exposure may affect different outcomes in males and females, warrant additional research on sexually dimorphic pathways.[20]

Limitations

Several limitations of this study should be noted. Firstly, the ECHO Cohort is drawn from several dozen existing longitudinal studies in an effort to establish a large national cohort with greater racial and geographic representation than can be accomplished by any single study. However, achieving this requires extensive efforts to harmonize constructs that were measured in slightly different ways and at a different times. To the extent that the effects of airborne lead exposure are specific to discrete cognitive processes, this approach may obscure the magnitude of the effect. Secondly, efforts to account for area-level confounders relied on census tract–level rather than individual-level data. Finally, these data can only address associations at the level of environmental exposure. Although it is expected that, on average, environmental exposure will correlate with actual biological absorption, data were not available on children's blood lead levels.

Public Health Implications

Environmental policies have typically sought to restrict lead concentrations with the expectation that exposure below a certain threshold has minimal effects. However, children are especially vulnerable to the neurotoxic effects of lead exposure, and even relatively minor insults to neurodevelopment are likely to accumulate over time. As such, airborne lead exposure likely contributes to disparities in children's cognitive development. In addition to direct efforts to reduce environmental pollution, attention to factors that may mitigate the impact of exposure on cognitive development, such as nutrition,[21] could reduce health disparities of lead exposure for vulnerable individuals. AJPH

ABOUT THE AUTHORS

Lisa M. Gatzke-Kopp is with the Department of Human Development and Family Studies, Pennsylvania State University, University Park. Michael Willoughby is with the Department of Education and Workforce Development, RTI International, Raleigh, NC. Amii M. Kress, Kristen McArthur, and Cara Wychgram are with the Department of General Epidemiology and Methodology, Johns Hopkins University, Baltimore, MD. David C. Folch is with the Department of Geography, Planning and Recreation, Northern Arizona University, Flagstaff. Steve Brunswasser is with the Department of Psychology, Rowan University, Glassboro, NJ. Dana Dabelea is with the Colorado School of Public Health, University of Colorado Anshutz Medical Campus, Aurora. Amy J. Elliott is with the Avera Research Institute, Sioux Falls, SD. Tina Hartert is with the Center for Health Services Research, Vanderbilt University, Nashville, TN. Margaret Karagas is with the Department of Epidemiology, Dartmouth Geisel School of Medicine, Lebanon, NH. Cindy T. McEvoy is with the Department of Pediatrics, Oregon Health Sciences University, Portland. James A. VanDerslice is with the Department of Public Health, University of Utah School of Medicine, Salt Lake City. Robert O. Wright and Rosalind J. Wright are with the Department of Pediatrics, Icahn School of Medicine at Mount Sinai, New York, NY.

CORRESPONDENCE

Correspondence should be sent to Lisa Gatzke-Kopp, Prevention Research Center, 315 BBH, Penn State, University Park, PA 16802 (e-mail: Lmk18@psu.edu). Reprints can be ordered at http://www.ajph.org by clicking the "Reprints" link.

PUBLICATION INFORMATION

Full Citation: Gatzke-Kopp LM, Willoughby M, Kress AM, et al. Airborne lead exposure and childhood cognition: the Environmental Influences on Child Health Outcomes (ECHO) cohort (2003–2022). *Am J Public Health*. 2024;114(3): 309–318.

Acceptance Date: October 27, 2023.

DOI: https://doi.org/10.2105/AJPH.2023.307519

ORCID iDs:
Lisa M. Gatzke-Kopp https://orcid.org/0000-0003-4470-4555

CONTRIBUTORS

L. M. Gatzke-Kopp, M. Willoughby, and D. C. Folch generated the original concept design with input from the project writing team: S. Brunswasser, D. Dabelea, A. J. Elliott, T. Hartert, M. Karagas, C. T. McEvoy, J. A. VanDerslice, R. O. Wright, and R. J. Wright. M. Willoughy, D. C. Folch, A. M. Kress, C. Wychgram, K. McArthur, and L. M. Gatzke-Kopp conducted analyses and interpreted the data. All authors contributed to the original manuscript draft and approval of the final version.

ACKNOWLEDGMENTS

Research reported in this publication was supported by the Environmental Influences on Child Health Outcomes (ECHO) Program, Office of the Director, National Institutes of Health, under award numbers U2COD023375 (Coordinating Center), U24OD023382 (Data Analysis Center), U24OD023319 with co-funding from the Office of Behavioral and Social Science Research (PRO Core), UH3OD023332 (L. M. G-K.; M. Swingler; L. Trasande), UH3OD023248 (D. D.), UH3OD023313 (S. Deoni; D. Koinis Mitchell), UH3OD023279 (A. J. E.), UH3OD023289 (A. Ferrara), UH3OD023282 (J. Gern), UH3OD023275 (M. K.), UH3OD023271 (C. Karr), UH3OD023347 (B. Lester), UH3OD023288 (C. T. M.), and UH3OD023337 (R. J. W., R. O. W.).

We thank our ECHO colleagues; the medical, nursing, and program staff; and the children and families participating in the ECHO cohorts. We also acknowledge the contribution of the following ECHO Program collaborators: ECHO Components—Coordinating Center: Duke Clinical Research Institute, Durham, NC: P. B. Smith, L. K. Newby; Data Analysis Center: Johns Hopkins University Bloomberg School of Public Health, Baltimore, MD: L. P. Jacobson; Research Triangle Institute, Durham, NC: D. J. Catellier; Person-Reported Outcomes Core: Northwestern University, Evanston, IL: R. Gershon, D. Cella. ECHO Awardees and Cohorts—Rhode Island Hospital, Providence: D. Koinis Mitchell; Rhode Island Hospital, Providence: S. Deoni, V. D'Sa; Kaiser Permanente Northern California Division of Research, Oakland: A. A. Ferrara; Kaiser Permanente Northern California Division of Research, Oakland: L. Croen; University of Wisconsin, Madison: J. Gern; University of Washington, Department of Environmental and Occupational Health Sciences, Seattle: C. Karr; University of Tennessee Health Science Center, Memphis: F. Tylavsky, A. Mason, Q. Zhao; Seattle Children's Research Institute, Seattle, WA: S. Sathyanarayana; University of California, San Francisco: N. Bush, K. Z. LeWinn; Women & Infants

Hospital of Rhode Island, Providence: B. Lester; Children's Mercy, Kansas City, MO: B. Carter; Corewell Health, Helen DeVos Children's Hospital, Grand Rapids, MI: S. Pastyrnak; Kapiolani Medical Center for Women and Children, Providence, RI: C. Neal; Los Angeles Biomedical Research Institute at Harbour-UCLA Medical Center, Los Angeles, CA: L. Smith; Wake Forest University School of Medicine, Winston Salem, NC: J. Helderman; Indiana University, Riley Hospital for Children, Indianapolis, IN: R. Tepper; Boston Children's Hospital, Boston, MA: M. Bosquet-Enlow; George Mason University, Fairfax, VA: K. Huddleston; New York University Grossman School of Medicine, New York, NY: L. Trasande; University of Minnesota, Minneapolis: R. Nguyen; University of Rochester Medical Center, Rochester, NY: E. Barrett; Icahn School of Medicine at Mount Sinai, New York, NY: S. Swan.

Note. The contents presented here are solely the responsibility of the authors and do not necessarily represent the official views of the National Institutes of Health.

CONFLICTS OF INTEREST

The authors have no conflicts of interest to disclose.

HUMAN PARTICIPANT PROTECTION

All participants provided written informed consent to the sharing of their archival data with the ECHO-wide data platform. The work of the ECHO Data Analysis Center is approved through the Johns Hopkins Bloomberg School of Public Health institutional review board.

REFERENCES

1. Wu Y, Sun J, Wang M, Yu G, Yu L, Wang C. The relationship of children's intelligence quotients and blood lead and zinc levels: a meta-analysis and system review. *Biol Trace Elem Res.* 2018; 182(2):185–195. https://doi.org/10.1007/s12011-017-1093-0
2. Collin MS, Venkatraman SK, Naveensubramaniam V, et al. Bioaccumulation of lead (Pb) and its effects on human: a review. *J Hazard Mater Adv.* 2022;7:100094. https://doi.org/10.1016/j.hazadv.2022.100094
3. Singh G, Singh V, Sobolewski M, Cory-Slechta D, Schneider JS. Sex-dependent effects of developmental lead exposure on the brain. *Front Genet.* 2018;9:89. https://doi.org/10.3389/fgene.2018.00089
4. Dignam T, Kaufmann RB, LeStourgeon L, Brown MJ. Control of lead sources in the United States, 1970–2017: public health progress and current challenges to eliminating lead exposure. *J Public Health Manag Pract.* 2019;25(suppl 1):S13–S22. https://doi.org/10.1097/PHH.0000000000000889
5. Grant LD. Lead and compounds. In: Lippmann M, Leikauf GD, eds. *Environmental Toxicants: Human Exposures and Their Health Effects.* 4th ed. New York, NY: Wiley; 2020:627–675. https://doi.org/10.1002/9781119438922.ch17
6. Hanna-Attisha M, LaChance J, Sadler RC, Schnepp AC. Elevated blood lead levels in children associated with the Flint drinking water crisis: a spatial analysis of risk and public health response. *Am J Public Health.* 2016;106(2): 283–290. https://doi.org/10.2105/AJPH.2015.303003
7. Jacobs DE. Lead-based paint as a major source of childhood lead poisoning: a review of the evidence. In: Beard ME, Iska SDA, eds. *Lead in Paint, Soil and Dust: Heath Risks, Exposure Studies, Control Measures, Measurement Methods, and Quality Assurance.* Philadelphia, PA: American Society for Testing and Materials; 1995:175–187. https://doi.org/10.1520/STP12974S
8. Gatzke-Kopp LM, Warkentien S, Willoughby M, et al. Proximity to sources of airborne lead is associated with reductions in children's executive function in the first four years of life. *Health Place.* 2021;68:102517. https://doi.org/10.1016/j.healthplace.2021.102517
9. Canfield RL, Jusko TA, Radegonde V. Airborne particulate lead and children's mental functioning. *Neurotoxicology.* 2020;81:288–293. https://doi.org/10.1016/j.neuro.2020.09.019
10. Knapp EA, Kress AM, Parker CB, et al. The Environmental influences on Child Health Outcomes (ECHO)-wide Cohort. *Am J Epidemiol.* 2023;192(8):1249–1263. https://doi.org/10.1093/aje/kwad071
11. Environmental Protection Agency. RSEI version 2.3.10. Available at: https://www.epa.gov/rsei/rsei-geographic-microdata-rsei-gm. Accessed May 2022.
12. Wechsler D. *Wechsler Adult Intelligence Scale–Third Edition: Administration and Scoring Manual.* San Antonio, TX: Psychological Corporation; 1997.
13. NIH toolbox for assessment of neurological and behavioral function: administrator's manual, 2006–2020. Version 1.17. National Institutes of Health and Northwestern University. Available at: https://www.google.com/url?sa=t&rct=j&q=&esrc=s&source=web&cd=&ved=2ahUKEwiftZzH9-mDAxUSk4kEHYclATwQFnoECCAQAQ&url=https%3A%2F%2Fwww.healthmeasures.net%2Fimages%2Fnihtoolbox%2FTraining-Admin-Scoring_Manuals%2FNIH_Toolbox_App_Administrators_Manual_v1.17.pdf&usg=AOvVaw12fmc4-24el_0BSMjVivpq&opi=89978449. Accessed January 22, 2024.
14. NIH toolbox scoring and interpretation guide for the iPad, 2021. National Institutes of Health and Northwestern University. Available at: https://www.google.com/url?sa=t&rct=j&q=&esrc=s&source=web&cd=&ved=2ahUKEwjiyrbw9umDAxUglokEHSmTBNkQFnoECBQQAQ&url=https%3A%2F%2Fwww.nihtoolbox.org%2Fapp%2Fuploads%2F2022%2F05%2FToolbox_Scoring_and_Interpretation_Guide_for_iPad_v1.7-5.25.21.pdf&usg=AOvVaw3zfK_Nxb2JcCXL-8RDmVB6&opi=89978449. Accessed January 22, 2024.
15. Rural Health Research Center Web site. Available at: https://depts.washington.edu/uwruca/ruca-uses.php. Accessed May 2022.
16. American Community Survey. Available at: https://www2.census.gov/programs-surveys/acs/summary_file/2009/data/5_year_entire_sf; https://www2.census.gov/programs-surveys/acs/summary_file/2014/data/5_year_entire_sf; https://www2.census.gov/programs-surveys/acs/summary_file/2019/data/5_year_entire_sf. Accessed May 2022.
17. Stuart EA, Azur M, Frangakis C, Leaf P. Multiple imputation with large data sets: a case study of the Children's Mental Health Initiative. *Am J Epidemiol.* 2009;169(9):1133–1139. https://doi.org/10.1093/aje/kwp026
18. Lanphear BP, Hornung R, Khoury J, et al. Low-level environmental lead exposure and children's intellectual function: an international pooled analysis. *Environ Health Perspect.* 2005;113(7): 894–899. https://doi.org/10.1289/ehp.7688
19. DiPietro JA, Voegtline KM. The gestational foundation of sex differences in development and vulnerability. *Neuroscience.* 2017;342:4–20. https://doi.org/10.1016/j.neuroscience.2015.07.068
20. Zhou C-C, He Y-Q, Gao Z-Y, Qu M-Q, Yan C-H. Sex differences in the effects of lead exposure on growth and development in young children. *Chemosphere.* 2020;250:126294. https://doi.org/10.1016/j.chemosphere.2020.126294
21. Ji Y, Hong X, Wang G, et al. A prospective birth cohort study on early childhood lead levels and attention deficit hyperactivity disorder: new insight on sex differences. *J Pediatr.* 2018;199: 124–131. https://doi.org/10.1016/j.jpeds.2018.03.076

Suicide Methods and Trends Across Race/Ethnicity, Age, and Sex Groups in Chicago, Illinois, 2015–2021

Janelle R. Goodwill, MSW, PhD, and Rachel Baccile, MPP

Objectives. To measure differences in suicide rates across race/ethnicity, age, and sex groups in Chicago, Illinois, from 2015 to 2021.

Methods. We calculated the incidence rate and annual percentage change in suicides among Asian, Black, Latino/a, and White persons in Chicago. We also analyzed patterns in suicide method across race/ethnicity, age, and sex groups.

Results. Suicides increased significantly among Black males (incidence rate ratio [IRR] = 1.10; 95% confidence interval [CI] = 1.01, 1.20), Black females (IRR = 1.18; 95% CI = 1.04, 1.33), and Latino males (IRR = 1.23; 95% CI = 1.11, 1.38) between 2015 and 2021. Suicides decreased overall among White Chicagoans during this period. A significantly greater proportion of Black males than Black females died by suicide using a firearm (55.79% vs 24.05%; $P < .001$). Similar results were detected for Latino males and females (32.99% vs 9.09%; $P = .001$) and White males and females (30.10% vs 11.73%; $P < .001$).

Conclusions. Black persons in Chicago were the only group to experience significant increases in suicide among both males and females from 2015 to 2021, although specific methods used varied by race/ethnicity and sex group. (*Am J Public Health*. 2024;114(3):319–328. https://doi.org/10.2105/AJPH.2023.307511)

AJPH March 2024, Vol. 114, No. 3

Violence in Chicago, Illinois, has been the source of much sociological inquiry and political debate. Educators, legislators, researchers, and local activists have spent decades working to identify systemic and environmental factors that can be leveraged to reduce and ultimately eradicate violence and crime in this city.[1–11] Despite these vital contributions and critical efforts, suicide persists as a form of self-inflicted violence that has gone sorely understudied in Chicago-focused violence prevention research.[12] National news outlets continue to highlight issues of homicide in Chicago but have yet to carefully consider how suicide also serves as a pervasive form of violence that is worthy of national attention and concern. Commentaries on homicide in Chicago abound, whereas queries that directly address suicide in Chicago remain scant. This oversight in recognizing both homicide and suicide as urgent priorities for violence prevention is disheartening and underscores the important work of Chicago journalists and reporters who have been diligent in their efforts to draw attention to the alarming increase in local suicides.[13–15]

National data indicate that the odds of past-year suicide attempt are greater for Black adults in the United States,[16] that suicide rates have increased among Black youths in recent years,[17] and that rates of suicide increased among Native American/Alaska Native, Hispanic/Latino/a, and Black Americans during the COVID-19 pandemic.[18,19] However, there has yet to be an investigation of suicide in Chicago that measures differences in both methods and trends. In an effort to redress this knowledge gap, we explored changes in suicide rates in Chicago between 2015 and 2021. We built on the initial work of journalist Lakeidra Chavis, who in 2020 was the first to report increases in suicide for Black persons in Cook County, Illinois.[13] Moreover, we probed for within-group differences to determine whether suicide method or rates varied by race/ethnicity, sex, and age.

METHODS

We conducted a descriptive cohort study of suicides in Chicago between January 1, 2015 and December 31, 2021. We downloaded death records from the Cook County Medical Examiner's Office Case Archive.[20] This office is responsible for determining the cause and manner of death for all deaths occurring in Cook County. The Medical Examiner's Office determined decedent age, sex, and race, and decedents' next of kin indicated ethnicity. We limited our analysis to deaths occurring in the city of Chicago only. We used population estimates from the American Community Survey years 2015 to 2021, which we accessed using the tidycensus[21] R package version 1.3.1. We calculated age-specific incidence rates of death by suicide per year by age, sex, and race/ethnicity. We also calculated age-standardized rates per year by sex and racial/ethnic group using the 2000 US standard population.[22] We present all incidence rates as deaths per 100 000 persons.

We categorized the sample by sex (male or female) and race (non-Latino/a Black, non-Latino/a White, or non-Latino/a Asian) or ethnicity (Latino/a). We estimated a Poisson regression model with the age-standardized count of deaths by suicide as the dependent variable. The independent variables included the calendar year and the log of the group population. The incidence rate ratio (IRR) represents the average annual change in the death by suicide rate during the study period (2015–2021). In additional analyses, we estimated the age-specific trends by sex and race/ethnicity. We constructed age groups based on groupings available in American Community Survey population estimates (5–14, 15–19, 20–24, 25–29, 30–34, 35–44, 45–64, and ≥ 65 years). We modeled overdispersed subgroups with a negative binomial regression rather than Poisson. We calculated robust 95% confidence intervals (CIs) with the sandwich R package version 3.0.[23] Given the few years of data available, we did not adjust for multiple comparisons to avoid increasing type II error and potentially missing important findings.[24]

Furthermore, we also probed for suicide method—or how individuals died. We coded categorical descriptions and counted frequencies both within and across groups. We tested differences using a χ^2 or Fisher's exact test. We used Stata version 17[25] and R version 4.2.2[26] for analyses.

RESULTS

When examining differences in suicide method by race/ethnicity and sex, we found that a significantly greater proportion of Black, Latino, and White males died by suicide using firearms relative to females in their same racial or ethnic group (Table 1). Black, Latina, and White females were significantly more likely to die by suicide via toxicity, overdose, or poisoning than were their male counterparts. No within-group sex differences emerged among Asian males and females in Chicago. Results also revealed that hanging or suffocation was the most common suicide method used by Black females (29.11%), Asian males (46.81%), Asian females (48.39%), Latino males (50.76%), Latina females (60%), White males (35.92%), and White females (41.84%). More than 55% of Black males in Chicago, however, died by suicide using a firearm (Table 1), making self-inflicted gunshot wounds the primary suicide method for Black males in this city.

Additional within-group comparisons revealed that among Asian Chicagoans, blunt force injuries (e.g., bodily trauma resulting from jumping or falling from heights, being struck by a train, or self-inflicted wounds) served as the second most common suicide method, followed by self-inflicted gunshot wound and overdose (Table 1). For Black individuals in Chicago, hanging or suffocation was the second most common method among males (22.11%), whereas toxicity, overdose, or poisoning was the second most common method for females (26.58%). Similar patterns were detected among Latino/a and White suicide decedents in Chicago. Less common suicide methods across groups included thermal injuries or immolation and drowning.

Descriptive analyses suggest that there are variations in age ranges across groups as well (Table 2). Asian and White decedents skewed older, with a mean age of 42.4 and 47.5 years, respectively, whereas Black and Latino/a decedents had a mean age of 37.6 and 37.9 years, respectively. There was also a greater proportion of Black (10.4%) and Latino/a (7.8%) children and adolescents younger than 20 years who died by suicide. Notably, the youngest person to die by suicide in Chicago was an 8-year-old Black male.

We found a statistically significant increase in the age-standardized death by suicide rate among Asian females (Table 3; Figure 1), with the age-standardized rate increasing from 3.5 in 2015 to 5.9 in 2021 (IRR = 1.12; 95% CI = 1.01, 1.24). As a result of an apparent change in slope in 2018, we tested for a breakpoint using the Davies test, but the results did not show

TABLE 1— Suicide Method by Race/Ethnicity and Sex of Persons Who Died by Suicide in Chicago, IL: 2015–2021

	Asian (n = 78)				Black (n = 364)				Latino/a (n = 252)				White (n = 814)			
	All, %	Male (n = 47), %	Female (n = 31), %	P	All, %	Male (n = 285), %	Female (n = 79), %	P	All, %	Male (n = 197), %	Female (n = 55), %	P	All, %	Male (n = 618), %	Female (n = 196), %	P
Suicide method																
Gunshot wound	9.0	8.5	9.7	> .99	48.9	55.8	24.1	< .001	27.8	33.0	9.1	< .001	25.7	30.1	11.7	< .001
Toxicity, overdose, or poisoning	7.7	6.4	9.7	.68	10.7	6.3	26.6	< .001	7.9	5.1	18.2	.001	13.3	10.4	22.5	< .001
Blunt force injuries	32.1	34.0	29.0	.64	14.0	13.0	17.7	.28	9.1	9.1	9.1	> .99	22.0	22.0	21.9	.98
Hanging/ suffocation	47.4	46.8	48.4	.89	23.6	22.1	29.1	.19	52.8	50.8	60.0	.23	37.4	35.9	41.8	.14
Drowning	3.9	4.3	3.2	> .99	2.2	2.1	2.5	> .99	1.6	1.5	1.8	> .99	1.1	0.8	2.0	.23
Thermal injuries/ immolation	...	...	...	...	0.6	0.7	...	> .99	0.8	0.5	1.8	.39	0.6	0.8	...	.6

significance ($P = .40$). This overall trend was likely driven by Asian females aged 20 to 24 years (IRR = 1.97; 95% CI = 1.05, 3.72) and aged 25 to 29 years (IRR = 1.98; 95% CI = 1.56, 2.53; Table 3). We did not detect a statistically significant trend among Asian males overall or in any age group (Table 3; Figure 1).

We also found a statistically significant increase in the age-standardized death by suicide rate among Black males, from 7.7 in 2015 to 14.1 in 2021 (IRR = 1.09; 95% CI = 1.04, 1.15), and Black females, from 1.5 in 2015 to 4.8 in 2021 (IRR = 1.19; 95% CI = 1.16, 1.23; Table 3, Figure 1). We also saw a significant positive trend in both Black male and female adolescents aged 15 to 19 years. Black females aged 65 years and older also had a significant increasing trend, whereas Black men aged 35 to 44 years had a significant decreasing trend. Black individuals in Chicago were the only racial/ethnic group to experience significant increases in suicide among both males and females during this period (Table 3; Figure 1).

The age-standardized death by suicide rate increased overall for Latino males (IRR = 1.24; 95% CI = 1.05, 1.48; Table 3). The majority of this increase occurred in 1 year, from 2015 to 2016, with the rate increasing from 0.7 to 6.3, an 8 times increase. By 2021, the rate had further increased to 10.4, and the trend remained statistically significant for just 2016 to 2021 (IRR = 1.10; 95% CI = 1.07, 1.14). The increase among Latino males appears to be driven by those aged 20 to 24 and 25 to 29 years as well as those aged 45 to 65 years. However, no statistically significant trend emerged for Latina females overall or across different age groups (Table 3).

Overall, age-standardized suicide rates trended downward from 2015 to 2021 among White persons in Chicago,

TABLE 2— Crude Count of Deaths by Suicide in Chicago, IL, by Sex, Race/Ethnicity, and Age Group: 2015–2021

	Asian			Black			Latino/a			White		
	All	Male	Female	All	Male	Female	All	Male	Female	All	Male	Female
Age groups, y, no. (%)												
All	78	47	31	367	286	81	254	199	55	826	629	197
5–14	0 (0.0)	0 (0)	0 (0)	11 (3.0)	6 (2.1)	5 (6.2)	9 (3.5)	3 (1.5)	6 (10.9)	3 (0.4)	1 (0.2)	2 (1.0)
15–19	2 (2.6)	1 (2.1)	1 (3.2)	27 (7.4)	21 (7.3)	6 (7.4)	11 (4.3)	8 (4.0)	3 (5.5)	18 (2.2)	13 (2.1)	5 (2.5)
20–24	8 (10.3)	6 (12.8)	2 (6.5)	58 (15.8)	49 (17.1)	9 (11.1)	42 (16.5)	33 (16.6)	9 (16.4)	61 (7.4)	47 (7.5)	14 (7.1)
25–29	16 (20.5)	9 (19.1)	7 (22.6)	60 (16.3)	50 (17.5)	10 (12.3)	38 (15.0)	34 (17.1)	4 (7.3)	77 (9.3)	61 (9.7)	16 (8.1)
30–34	11 (14.1)	5 (10.6)	6 (19.4)	40 (10.9)	29 (10.1)	11 (13.6)	20 (7.9)	16 (8.0)	4 (7.3)	84 (10.2)	58 (9.2)	26 (13.2)
35–44	13 (16.7)	10 (21.3)	3 (9.7)	59 (16.1)	48 (16.8)	11 (13.6)	47 (18.5)	36 (18.1)	11 (20.0)	139 (16.8)	110 (17.5)	29 (14.7)
45–64	13 (16.7)	7 (14.9)	6 (19.4)	76 (20.7)	54 (18.9)	22 (27.2)	71 (28.0)	54 (27.1)	17 (30.9)	294 (35.6)	221 (35.1)	73 (37.1)
≥65	15 (19.2)	9 (19.1)	6 (19.4)	36 (9.8)	29 (10.1)	7 (8.6)	16 (6.3)	15 (7.5)	1 (1.8)	150 (18.2)	118 (18.8)	32 (16.2)
Age distribution, y												
Range	17–94	19–94	17–85	8–94	8–94	11–84	12–82	12–82	12–75	11–98	13–95	11–98
Mean (SD)	42.4 (18.8)	41.9 (18.7)	43.1 (19.2)	37.6 (17.7)	37.5 (18.0)	37.6 (16.8)	37.9 (16)	38.3 (15.8)	36.5 (16.8)	47.5 (17.9)	47.8 (17.9)	46.3 (17.7)
Median (IQR)	35 (28–58)	35 (27–54)	33 (28–59)	32 (24–49)	32 (24–48)	34 (25–50)	37 (25–44)	37 (25–49)	36 (22–51)	47 (32–60)	47 (21–61)	47 (31–58)

Note. IQR = interquartile range.

with the rate decreasing for males from 20.0 to 18.0 (IRR = 0.98; 95% CI = 0.96, 0.99) and for females from 6.4 to 4.8 (IRR = 0.96; 95% CI = 0.95, 0.98; Table 3; Figure 1). Within-group analyses of age differences indicated that suicide rates decreased significantly for White men aged 30 to 34 years and for White women aged 30 to 34 and 35 to 44 years (Table 3). White individuals in Chicago were the only group to experience decreases in suicide among both males and females throughout this 7-year time span.

DISCUSSION

Results yielded from this investigation offer a new contribution to the literature by first assessing both within- and across-racial/ethnic group differences in suicide rates in the city of Chicago—a popular location for ethnographic study yet an understudied city in the suicide prevention literature. We also measured patterns in suicide method as a means to more clearly ascertain mechanisms that exacerbate risk of death by suicide. Our evaluation confirms that suicides increased significantly among Black males and females and among Latino males between 2015 and 2021. Increases in suicide rates reflect both an increase in the number of deaths by suicide and a decrease in the population of Black and Latino/a Chicagoans.

We also learned that suffocation or hanging is the most common suicide method for most groups—with the exception of Black males, who most often ended their lives via a self-inflicted gunshot wound. Preventing suicide via hanging or suffocation is especially difficult in that several common household items can be used for suffocation. Scholars note that suicide via hanging or suffocation has increased over time in the

TABLE 3— Age-Standardized and Age-Specific IRRs of Change in Death by Suicide in Chicago, IL, by Sex, Race/Ethnicity, and Age Group: 2015–2021

Age Group	Asian, IRR (CI)		Black, IRR (CI)		Latino/a, IRR (CI)		White, IRR (CI)	
	Male	Female	Male	Female	Male	Female	Male	Female
Overall, age standardized	1.12 (0.94, 1.33)	1.12 (1.01, 1.24)	1.09 (1.04, 1.15)[a]	1.19 (1.16, 1.23)	1.24 (1.05, 1.48)[a]	1.07 (0.99, 1.16)	0.98 (0.96, 0.99)	0.96 (0.95, 0.98)
Overall	1.11 (0.98, 1.25)	1.19 (0.97, 1.47)	1.10 (1.01, 1.20)[a]	1.18 (1.02, 1.36)	1.23 (1.11, 1.38)[a]	1.06 (0.95, 1.19)	0.98 (0.93, 1.04)[a]	0.98 (0.91, 1.05)[a]
Aged 5–14 y	...	...	1.34 (0.85, 2.12)	1.14 (0.82,1.57)	...	1.41 (0.95, 2.09)	...	...
Aged 15–19 y	...	...	1.21 (1.09, 1.34)	1.77 (1.01, 3.12)	0.84 (0.46, 1.43)[a]	...	0.84 (0.7, 1.01)	1.05 (0.81, 1.37)
Aged 20–24 y	1.05 (0.77, 1.43)	1.97 (1.05, 3.72)	1.21 (1.11, 1.32)[a]	0.94 (0.72, 1.22)	1.27 (1.05, 0.54)	1.03 (0.74, 1.42)	1.03 (0.92, 1.15)	1.10 (0.84, 1.43)
Aged 25–29 y	1.04 (0.79, 1.36)	1.98 (1.56, 2.53)	1.10 (0.95, 1.27)[a]	1.34 (0.99, 1.82)	1.32 (1.18,1.48)	...	0.91 (0.83, 1.01)	0.95 (0.80, 1.14)
Aged 30–34 y	1.13 (0.86, 1.49)	1.09 (0.87, 1.38)	1.22 (1.18, 1.26)	1.08 (0.91, 1.28)	1.19 (0.95, 1.48)	...	0.92 (0.86, 0.97)	0.84 (0.75, 0.94)
Aged 35–44 y	1.20 (0.90, 1.58)	...	0.93 (0.87, 0.99)	1.16 (0.94, 1.44)	1.12 (0.93, 1.34)	1.03 (0.92, 1.16)	0.99 (1.03, 1.05)	0.87 (0.78, 0.98)
Aged 45–64 y	1.32 (0.89, 1.97)	1.11 (0.72, 1.71)	1.07 (0.95, 1.20)	1.13 (0.89, 1.43)	1.30 (1.16,1.46)	1.03 (0.83, 1.26)[a]	0.99 (0.93, 1.04)	1.01 (0.92, 1.11)
Aged ≥ 65 y	1.00 (0.72, 1.38)	...	1.01 (0.86, 1.17)	1.46 (1.01, 2.10)	1.14 (0.89, 1.46)	...	1.03 (0.95, 1.11)	1.08 (0.92, 1.27)

Note. CI = confidence interval; IRR = incidence rate ratio. Ellipses indicate too few observations to fit a model. Crude counts of deaths by race/ethnicity and sex can be found in Table 2. We estimated IRRs from coefficient on calendar year in regression models. All age group models included 5 observations, 1 for each year, with crude count of deaths and the population estimate. The overall and overall age-standardized models included 40 observations, 1 for each year + age group combination, with crude count of deaths and the population estimate.
[a]Negative binomial model used because of overdispersion.

United States,[27] yet there are only a few places where restrictions to potentially lethal means used for hanging or suffocation exist (e.g., hospitals, schools).[28] This ease of access will require interventionists and clinicians to continue developing behavioral interventions that are readily available to those in need, as there is no way to guarantee that individuals will be restricted from accessing potentially lethal items at all times and across all circumstances.[28]

Ultimately, our findings further complicate understandings of gun violence in Chicago by demonstrating that Black males in Chicago use guns to end their own lives more than any other racial/ethnic or sex group in the city. This finding aligns with previous work in this area,[29–32] and violence prevention initiatives must expand beyond homicide to also recognize suicide prevention as a necessary priority for promoting hope and healing for Black males. Illinois has already adopted gun laws that are stricter than those of other states, as evidenced by the Firearm Restraining Order that went into law in 2019 and calls for the removal of firearms from persons who may be at risk for harming themselves or other people.[33]

Another policy change, the Protect Illinois Communities Act, which bans the "sale and distribution of assault weapons, high-capacity magazines, and switches in Illinois,"[34] was signed into law by Governor Pritzker in January 2023. Still, discerning whether someone is at risk for suicide at the time of gun purchase is a more difficult feat.

One potential change would include updating the eligibility criteria for the Firearm Owners Identification card, as approval of this application is required before any Illinois resident is permitted to legally obtain and possess a firearm

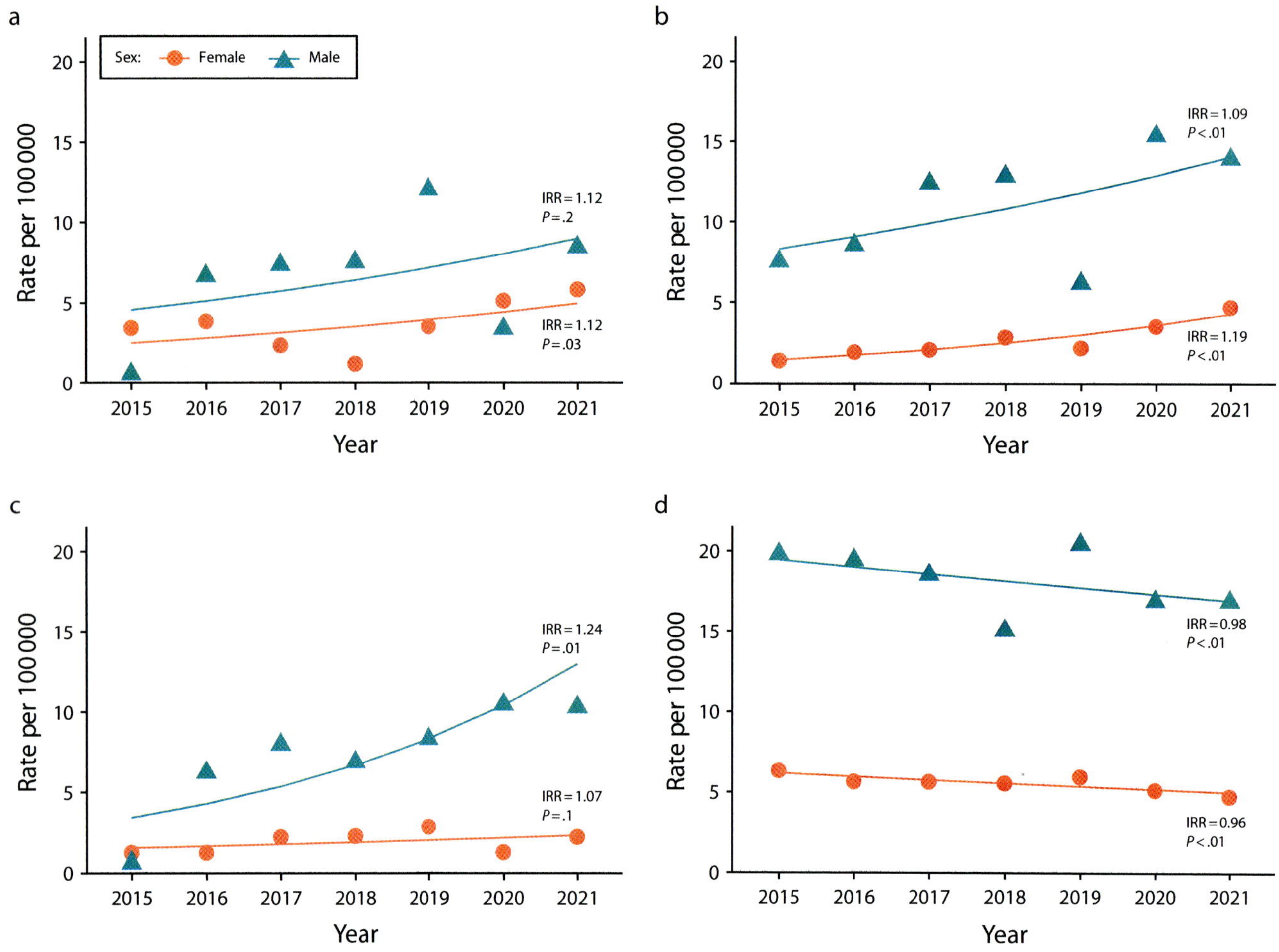

FIGURE 1— Age-Standardized Rate of Deaths by Suicide per 100 000 Persons in Chicago, IL, by Sex and Race/Ethnicity: 2015–2021

Note. IRR = incidence rate ratio.

or ammunition. The Firearm Owners Identification card application includes 15 eligibility criteria, and only 2 speak directly to issues of mental health or history of mental illness. None of the criteria address recent experiences of suicidality.[34] Thus, (1) adding eligibility criteria that confirm individuals are not currently suicidal, and (2) providing all applicants, irrespective of their current risk level, with suicide warning signs and prevention resources could prove fruitful in developing upstream interventions that may aid in preventing suicides across the city. Although there is no way for us to determine whether the persons who died by suicide via firearm did so using guns they were licensed to carry, we see the revision of Firearm Owners Identification card eligibility criteria and the dissemination of suicide prevention resources as noninvasive and low-cost strategies for potentially restricting access to firearms.

Our findings also align with a recent Centers for Disease Control and Prevention (CDC) report that found significant increases in suicides among Black, Hispanic, and Native American/Alaska Native groups during the COVID-19 pandemic.[18] National data indicate that suicides decreased among White Americans between 2018 and 2021.[18] Our results corroborate trends reported across other states[35] and at the national level,[18] as Black persons in Chicago were the only group to experience significant increases in suicides among both males and females, with suicides increasing 18% in Black females and 10% among Black males between 2015 and 2021. Rates of suicide remain highest for White Chicagoans relative to all other racial/ethnic groups in the city, yet White Chicagoans were the only group to experience statistically significant decreases in suicide for both males and females from 2015 to 2021. These differences in trends across racial/ethnic groups may be the result of disparities in access to affordable and adequate mental health treatment that existed before the pandemic.[36,37]

Furthermore, suicide rates increased among Asian women aged 20 to 29 years, pointing to the need to reach this group through interventions targeting young adults and college-aged or student populations. It is important to note that Asian Chicagoans were the smallest racial or ethnic group included in this analysis, which is likely a reflection of our intention to focus exclusively on suicides that occurred in the city of Chicago. Future studies should measure trends among Asian youths and young adults who live in suburbs or cities near Chicago, as their experiences and access to treatment may differ from those residing within city limits.

Moreover, suicides increased significantly for Black male adolescents and young adults, although suicide rates decreased for Black men aged 35 to 44 years. Suicides increased among Black females aged 15 to 19 years and among those aged 65 years and older (Table 3). The trend of Black males and females dying by suicide during adolescence and young adulthood reiterates the necessity of administering suicide prevention interventions early and often,[38–40] especially when considering that the youngest person to die by suicide in Chicago from 2015 to 2021 was an 8-year-old Black boy.

Earlier scholarship led by Bridge[41,42] and Sheftall[43] points to increased risk of suicide among elementary-aged and early adolescent Black children when compared with their White peers.[44] A recent analysis published by these authors confirms that similar trends continued during the COVID-19 pandemic, with suicides increasing significantly among Black and Native American/Alaska Native youths between March 1, 2020, and December 31, 2020.[45] Conversely, the finding that suicides increased for older Black females in Chicago is surprising and diverges from earlier studies that found that older Black men reported more ideation and attempts than did older Black women in a national sample.[46] Additional efforts are needed to more carefully assess the risk factors that uniquely contribute to suicide for Black Americans across the developmental life course.

Findings from Latino/a Chicagoans in this sample show significant increases in suicides among Latino males aged 20 to 29 and 45 to 64 years. These results partially align with current national trends, as recent CDC data confirm that suicides increased 19.4% among Latino/a adults aged 25 to 44 years between 2018 and 2021. Suicides did, however, decrease significantly in older Latino/a adults aged 45 to 64 years.[18] Researchers detected no significant changes in suicide trends among younger (e.g., 10–24-year-old) Latino/a youths in the United States.[18] Other studies of suicidality in Latino/a youths reveal that suicide attempts for this population are not significantly different from other ethnic groups[47,48] and that suicides did not increase among Latino/a adolescents during the earliest phase of the COVID-19 pandemic in 2020.[45] When taking our findings into account, it is evident that more work is needed to further disentangle within-group age differences in suicide risk for Latino/a communities during the COVID-19 pandemic.

Limitations

It is important to first note the limited time frame for which data were available. Our models included data from 2015 to 2021, so we cannot account for longer-term trends, and it is possible that observing differences over the course of 10 years or more would yield more stable or consistent findings over time. In light of the short study time frame, we assumed linear trends for all groups. However, this may not best fit all subgroup trends (e.g., Asian females). Future work with additional time points should consider segmented regression to describe changes in trends over time. Furthermore, we ran multiple statistical tests, and it is possible that some findings may be attributable to chance. These considerations are especially pertinent when conducting subgroup analyses with small samples (e.g., Asian males and females) for whom suicide was a rare event. Ultimately we did not correct significance thresholds for multiple comparisons, although future studies may consider doing so.

It is also important to consider that there were too few or no individuals listed as American Indian/Alaska Native, Multiracial, or Middle Eastern or North African who are recorded as dying by suicide in Chicago in the study time frame. Additionally, ethnicity classifications were limited for decedents who did not have next of kin willing or able to identify their ethnicity, and detailed information describing decedents' country of origin was not available for all persons. For example, categorization of the Latino/a ethnic group would benefit from collecting data that describe familial country of origin, as earlier studies have considered some of the unique suicide risk factors among Puerto Rican[49] and Mexican versus Cuban youths.[50] These same considerations are pertinent when working to understand the experiences of Black (e.g., African American vs Caribbean Black) and Asian (e.g., Chinese vs Korean) Americans as well, as both groups represent communities with robust ethnic diversity. Assessing intragroup differences could aid in developing culturally grounded interventions and treatment services for different groups and neighborhoods throughout Chicago.

Additionally, we did not distinguish differences between residents and nonresidents. Furthermore, it is plausible that some of the deaths categorized by the Medical Examiner's Office as overdoses may have been intentional suicides. Without a suicide note, it is difficult to tell. It will be beneficial for researchers to interrogate these matters in more detail moving forward. Data from the Cook County Medical Examiner's Office Case Archive also lacked information describing decedents' gender identity. A recent report from the Trevor Project found that among an online sample of more than 3000 Black and Multiracial Black LGBTQ (lesbian, gay, bisexual, transgender, queer or questioning) youths, more than half of transgender and nonbinary participants seriously considered suicide, with an additional 25% reporting an attempt in the past year.[51] Future suicidology research should continue to probe for within-group differences by working to ascertain pertinent risk and protective factors for Black Americans across varying age, gender, and ethnic groups.

Public Health Implications and Next Steps

Our analysis reveals both similarities and differences in suicide method across race/ethnicity and sex groups in Chicago, with most people turning to hanging or suffocation as a means to end their life. Study results also yield critical insights into current trends that reveal alarming increases in suicide among some of Chicago's most vulnerable groups. Together these findings disrupt national narratives about violence in Chicago by confirming that Black and Latino/a communities are at increased risk for dying by suicide, and not just homicide alone. Immediate efforts are therefore needed to curtail rising suicide rates by identifying mechanisms[52] that uniquely contribute to suicidality while also accounting for the structural and systemic barriers that prevent Chicagoans from receiving the mental health treatment they need.[53]

The Collaborative for Community Wellness—an interdisciplinary group of local mental health professionals and organizers—is leading critical efforts through the Treatment Not Trauma Campaign to fight for the reopening of Chicago's closed public mental health facilities and to promote nonpolice responses to mental health crises across the city.[54] Still, a great work remains ahead to ensure that all persons in Chicago have equitable access to mental health treatment that is safe, affordable, and accessible in their local communities. For these reasons, our next steps in this line of work include using spatial analysis to measure suicide rates across neighborhoods, with a particular focus on trends relative to closures of public mental health facilities—most of which occurred in neighborhoods located on the South and West sides of Chicago.[13,14,53] Such an endeavor not only will improve quality of life for members of historically marginalized groups but will also have direct implications for state and local policies that are implemented in the years to come. AJPH

ABOUT THE AUTHORS

Janelle R. Goodwill is with the University of Chicago Crown Family School of Social Work, Policy, and Practice, Chicago, IL. Rachel Baccile is with the University of Chicago Center for Health and the Social Sciences, Chicago.

CORRESPONDENCE

Correspondence should be sent to Janelle R. Goodwill, 969 E. 60th St, Chicago, IL 60637 (e-mail: jgoodwill@uchicago.edu). Reprints can be ordered at http://www.ajph.org by clicking the "Reprints" link.

PUBLICATION INFORMATION

Full Citation: Goodwill JR, Baccile R. Suicide methods and trends across race/ethnicity, age, and sex groups in Chicago, Illinois, 2015–2021. *Am J Public Health*. 2024;114(3):319–328.

Acceptance Date: October 21, 2023.

DOI: https://doi.org/10.2105/AJPH.2023.307511

ORCID iDs:
Janelle R. Goodwill https://orcid.org/0000-0001-9887-837X

CONTRIBUTORS

J. R. Goodwill conceptualized and designed the study. Both authors analyzed the data, drafted the article, and reviewed and approved the final version.

CONFLICTS OF INTEREST

The authors have no conflicts of interest to report.

HUMAN PARTICIPANT PROTECTION

This study did not meet the definition of human participant research, as this is a secondary analysis of data that are available to the public as determined by the University of Chicago Crown Family School of Social Work and Chapin Hall institutional review board.

REFERENCES

1. Bell CC, Jenkins EJ. Community violence and children on Chicago's Southside. *Psychiatry*. 1993;56(1):46–54. https://doi.org/10.1080/00332747.1993.11024620
2. Gaylord-Harden NK, So S, Bai GJ, Tolan PH. Examining the effects of emotional and cognitive desensitization to community violence exposure in male adolescents of color. *Am J Orthopsychiatry*. 2017;87(4):463–473. https://doi.org/10.1037/ort0000241
3. Mason M, McLone S, Monuteaux MC, Sheehan K, Lee LK, Fleegler EW. Association between youth homicides and state spending: a Chicago cross-sectional case study. *BMJ Open*. 2022;12(1):e052933. https://doi.org/10.1136/bmjopen-2021-052933
4. Green B, Horel T, Papachristos AV. Modeling contagion through social networks to explain

and predict gunshot violence in Chicago, 2006 to 2014. *JAMA Intern Med*. 2017;177(3):326–333. https://doi.org/10.1001/jamainternmed.2016.8245

5. Irsheid SB, Garthe RC, Gorman-Smith D, Schoeny M. The implications of executive functioning on community adversity and violence and mental health outcomes. *Youth Soc*. 2023;55(2):321–350. https://doi.org/10.1177/0044118X211053026
6. Voisin DR, Patel S, Hong JS, Takahashi L, Gaylord-Harden N. Behavioral health correlates of exposure to community violence among African-American adolescents in Chicago. *Child Youth Serv Rev*. 2016;69:97–105. https://doi.org/10.1016/j.childyouth.2016.08.006
7. Papachristos AV, Brazil N, Cheng T. Understanding the crime gap: violence and inequality in an American city. *City Community*. 2018;17(4):1051–1074. https://doi.org/10.1111/cico.12348
8. Sampson RJ, Wilson WJ. Toward a theory of race, crime, and urban inequality. In: Hagan J, Peterson R, eds. *Crime and Inequality*. Stanford, CA: Stanford University Press; 1995:37–54. https://doi.org/10.1515/9781503615557-004
9. Ralph L. *Renegade Dreams: Living Through Injury in Gangland Chicago*. Chicago, IL: University of Chicago Press; 2014.
10. Patton DU, Miller RJ, Garbarino J, Gale A, Kornfeld E. Hardiness scripts: high-achieving African American boys in a Chicago charter school navigating community violence and school. *J Community Psychol*. 2016;44(5):638–655. https://doi.org/10.1002/jcop.21791
11. Gorman-Smith D, Tolan PH. Positive adaptation among youth exposed to community violence. In: Luthar SS, ed. *Resilience and Vulnerability: Adaptation in the Context of Childhood Adversities*. Cambridge, UK: Cambridge University Press; 2003:392–413.
12. Stack S. Homicide followed by suicide: an analysis of Chicago data. *Criminology*. 1997;35(3):435–453. https://doi.org/10.1111/j.1745-9125.1997.tb01224.x
13. Chavis L. In Chicago, a steep rise in suicide among Black people. *The Trace*. June 25, 2020. Available at: https://www.thetrace.org/2020/07/in-chicago-a-steep-rise-in-suicide-among-black-people. Accessed August 10, 2020.
14. Chavis L. More suicides by Black Cook County residents in 2020 than in any year in over a decade. *Chicago Sun Times*. February 19, 2021. Available at: https://chicago.suntimes.com/2021/2/19/22290148/suicide-black-cook-county-residents-rise-mental-health-covid-coronavirus. Accessed February 22, 2021.
15. Hasan A. Data shows surge in suicides among Cook County's Black population. July 29, 2020. Available at: https://www.wbez.org/stories/data-shows-surge-in-suicides-among-cook-countys-black-population/7d548c96-cbfd-48dc-9d0d-fd4bbecf85dd. Accessed September 1, 2020.
16. Bommersbach TJ, Rosenheck RA, Rhee TG. National trends of mental health care among US adults who attempted suicide in the past 12 months. *JAMA Psychiatry*. 2022;79(3):219–231. https://doi.org/10.1001/jamapsychiatry.2021.3958
17. Sheftall AH, Vakil F, Ruch DA, Boyd RC, Lindsey MA, Bridge JA. Black youth suicide: investigation of current trends and precipitating circumstances. *J Am Acad Child Adolesc Psychiatry*. 2022;61(5):662–675. https://doi.org/10.1016/j.jaac.2021.08.021
18. Centers for Disease Control and Prevention. Notes from the field: recent changes in suicide rates, by race and ethnicity and age group—United States, 2021. *MMWR Morb Mortal Wkly Rep*. 2023;72(6):160–162. https://doi.org/10.15585/mmwr.mm7206a4
19. Goodwill JR. Purpose in the pandemic: fear of COVID-19, hopelessness, meaning in life, and suicidal thoughts among two samples of Black Americans. *Am Psychol*. 2023;78(6):775–789. https://doi.org/10.1037/amp0001171
20. Cook County Medical Examiner. Medical Examiner Case Archive. January 13, 2024. Available at: https://datacatalog.cookcountyil.gov/Public-Safety/Medical-Examiner-Case-Archive/cjeq-bs86. Accessed January 13, 2022.
21. Walker K, Herman M, Eberwein K. tidycensus. September 16, 2023. Available at: https://cran.r-project.org/web/packages/tidycensus/index.html. Accessed January 12, 2024.
22. National Cancer Institute. Standard populations—single ages: surveillance, epidemiology, and end results. Available at: https://seer.cancer.gov/stdpopulations. Accessed January 12, 2024.
23. Zeileis A, Köll S, Graham N. Various versatile variances: an object-oriented implementation of clustered covariances in R. *J Stat Softw*. 2020;95(1):1–36. https://doi.org/10.18637/jss.v095.i01
24. Rothman KJ. No adjustments are needed for multiple comparisons. *Epidemiology*. 1990;1(1):43–46. https://doi.org/10.1097/00001648-199001000-00010
25. StataCorp. *Stata Statistical Software, Release 16*. [computer program]. College Station, TX: StataCorp LP; 2019.
26. R Foundation. The R Project for Statistical Computing. Available at: https://www.r-project.org. Accessed January 12, 2024.
27. Baker SP, Hu G, Wilcox HC, Baker TD. Increase in suicide by hanging/suffocation in the U.S., 2000–2010. *Am J Prev Med*. 2013;44(2):146–149. https://doi.org/10.1016/j.amepre.2012.10.010
28. Gunnell D, Bennewith O, Hawton K, Simkin S, Kapur N. The epidemiology and prevention of suicide by hanging: a systematic review. *Int J Epidemiol*. 2005;34(2):433–442. https://doi.org/10.1093/ije/dyh398
29. Joe S, Kaplan MS. Firearm-related suicide among young African-American males. *Psychiatr Serv*. 2002;53(3):332–334. https://doi.org/10.1176/appi.ps.53.3.332
30. Joe S, Kaplan MS. Suicide among African American men. *Suicide Life Threat Behav*. 2001;(31 suppl):106–121. https://doi.org/10.1521/suli.31.1.5.106.24223
31. Gibbs JT. African-American suicide: a cultural paradox. *Suicide Life Threat Behav*. 1997;27(1):68–79. https://doi.org/10.1111/j.1943-278X.1997.tb00504.x
32. Cubbage J, Adams L. Still ringing the alarm: an enduring call to action for Black youth suicide prevention. August 23, 2023. Available at: https://publichealth.jhu.edu/sites/default/files/2023-08/2023-august-still-ringing-alarm.pdf. Accessed January 13, 2024.
33. Gatens A. Firearm restraining orders in Illinois. March 11, 2022. Available at: https://icjia.illinois.gov/researchhub/articles/firearm-restraining-orders-in-illinois. Accessed January 13, 2024.
34. Illinois State Police. Firearm owners identification (FOID). 2023. Available at: https://isp.illinois.gov/Foid/Foid. Accessed July 5, 2023.
35. Bray MJC, Daneshvari NO, Radhakrishnan I, et al. Racial differences in statewide suicide mortality trends in Maryland during the Coronavirus disease 2019 (COVID-19) pandemic. *JAMA Psychiatry*. 2021;78(4):444–446. https://doi.org/10.1001/jamapsychiatry.2020.3938
36. Snowden LR. Barriers to effective mental health services for African Americans. *Ment Health Serv Res*. 2001;3(4):181–187. https://doi.org/10.1023/a:1013172913880
37. Planey AM, Smith SMN, Moore S, Walker TD. Barriers and facilitators to mental health help-seeking among African American youth and their families: a systematic review study. *Child Youth Serv Rev*. 2019;101:190–200. https://doi.org/10.1016/j.childyouth.2019.04.001
38. Robinson WLV, Whipple CR, Keenan K, Flack CE, Wingate LR. Suicide in African American adolescents: understanding risk by studying resilience. *Annu Rev Clin Psychol*. 2022;18:359–385. https://doi.org/10.1146/annurev-clinpsy-072220-021819
39. Goodwill JR, Yasui M. Mental health service utilization, school experiences, and religious involvement among a national sample of Black adolescents who attempted suicide: examining within and cross-race group differences. *Child Adolesc Soc Work J*. [Published October 14, 2022]. https://doi.org/10.1007/s10560-022-00888-8
40. Brooks JR, Madubata IJ, Jewell RD, Ortiz DA, Walker RL. Depression and suicide ideation: the role of self-acceptance for Black young adults. *J Black Psychol*. 2023;49(3):382–403. https://doi.org/10.1177/00957984211037440
41. Bridge JA, Asti L, Horowitz LM, et al. Suicide trends among elementary school-aged children in the United States from 1993 to 2012. *JAMA Pediatr*. 2015;169(7):673–677. https://doi.org/10.1001/jamapediatrics.2015.0465
42. Bridge JA, Horowitz LM, Fontanella CA, et al. Age-related racial disparity in suicide rates among US youths from 2001 through 2015. *JAMA Pediatr*. 2018;172(7):697–699. https://doi.org/10.1001/jamapediatrics.2018.0399
43. Sheftall AH, Asti L, Horowitz LM, et al. Suicide in elementary school-aged children and early adolescents. *Pediatrics*. 2016;138(4):e20160436. https://doi.org/10.1542/peds.2016-0436
44. Opara I, Assan MA, Pierre K, et al. Suicide among Black children: an integrated model of the interpersonal-psychological theory of suicide and intersectionality theory for researchers and clinicians. *J Black Stud*. 2020;51(6):611–631. https://doi.org/10.1177/0021934720935641
45. Bridge JA, Ruch DA, Sheftall AH, et al. Youth suicide during the first year of the COVID-19 pandemic. *Pediatrics*. 2023;151(3):e2022058375. https://doi.org/10.1542/peds.2022-058375
46. Joe S, Ford BC, Taylor RJ, Chatters LM. Prevalence of suicide ideation and attempts among Black Americans in later life. *Transcult Psychiatry*. 2014;51(2):190–208. https://doi.org/10.1177/1363461513503381
47. Centers for Disease Control and Prevention. Suicidal ideation and behaviors among high school students—Youth Risk Behavior Survey, United

States, 2019. *MMWR Suppl.* 2020;69(1):47–55. https://doi.org/10.15585/mmwr.su6901a6

48. Lindsey MA, Sheftall AH, Xiao Y, Joe S. Trends of suicidal behaviors among high school students in the United States: 1991–2017. *Pediatrics.* 2019;144(5):e20191187. https://doi.org/10.1542/peds.2019-1187
49. Polanco-Roman L, Alvarez K, Corbeil T, et al. Association of childhood adversities with suicide ideation and attempts in Puerto Rican young adults. *JAMA Psychiatry.* 2021;78(8):896–902. https://doi.org/10.1001/jamapsychiatry.2021.0480
50. Vélez-Grau C, Lindsey MA. Do connectedness and self-esteem play a role in the transition to future suicide attempts among Latina and Latino youth with suicide ideation? *Child Youth Serv Rev.* 2022;139(106553):106553. https://doi.org/10.1016/j.childyouth.2022.106553
51. Trevor Project. Mental health of Black transgender and nonbinary young people. February 2023. Available at: https://www.thetrevorproject.org/wp-content/uploads/2023/02/EMBARGOED_2.28.23_The-Trevor-Project-Research-Brief_Black-TGNB-Youth-Mental-Health.pdf. Accessed January 12, 2024.
52. Goodwill JR. Reasons for suicide in Black young adults: a latent class analysis. *J Racial Ethn Health Disparities.* 2024;11(1):425–440. https://doi.org/10.1007/s40615-023-01530-8
53. Moreno N. Closing the gap: how the 2012 mental health clinic closures hurt Chicagoans. March 10, 2021. Available at: https://www.wbez.org/stories/closing-the-gap-how-the-2012-mental-health-clinic-closures-hurt-chicagoans/0c4bc618-2470-41a6-8c1d-d74f7bbe26c9. Accessed May 1, 2023.
54. Collaborative for Community Wellness. Treatment not trauma: a community care infrastructure for crisis response, mental health, and shared safety. July 2023. Available at: https://www.collaborativeforcommunitywellness.org/_files/ugd/c29cfd_fab7be98357d4fbd9bbdb833698284c7.pdf. September 18, 2023.

Salary Disparities in Public Health Occupations: Analysis of Federal Data, 2021–2022

Heather Krasna, PhD, EdM, MS, Malvika Venkataraman, MS, and Isabella Patino, BA

See also Resnick et al. p. 264.

Objectives. To assess salary differences between workers within key public health occupations in local or state government and workers in the same occupations in the private sector.

Methods. We used the US Department of Labor's Occupational Employment and Wage Survey (OEWS). Referencing previous studies matching Standard Occupational Classification (SOC) codes with health department occupations, we selected 44 SOC codes. We contrasted median salaries in OEWS for workers in each occupation within state or local government with workers in the same occupations outside government.

Results. Thirty of 44 occupations paid at least 5% less in government than the private sector, with 10 occupations, primarily in management, computer, and scientific or research occupations paying between 20% and 46.9% less in government. Inspection and compliance roles, technicians, and certain clinicians had disparities of 10% to 19%. Six occupations, primarily in social work or counseling, paid 24% to 38.7% more in government.

Conclusions. To develop a sustainable public health workforce, health departments must consider adjusting their salaries if possible, market their strong benefits or public service mission, or use creative recruitment incentives such as student loan repayment programs for hard-to-fill roles.
(*Am J Public Health*. 2024;114(3):329–339. https://doi.org/10.2105/AJPH.2023.307512)

AJPH March 2024, Vol. 114, No. 3

The local, state, tribal, and territorial government public health departments (HDs)[1,2] in the United States serve as our nation's frontline defense against disease but are severely understaffed,[2] with studies documenting workforce shortages, recruitment challenges, and pay inequity for key occupations such as epidemiologists[3,4] and public health nurses,[5–7] and labor market competition for public health degree graduates.[8] While factors such as job satisfaction, public service motivation,[9] flexible schedules, or benefits can attract candidates to apply for jobs, salary is known to be paramount in recruitment competition, including in public health.[3,8,10,11] According to the Public Health Workforce Interests and Needs Survey (PH WINS), three quarters of HD staff aged 35 years or younger quit between 2017 and 2021, and pay was the most commonly cited reason for considering leaving their role (63%).[2] Generally, salary is a key recruitment and retention factor; a national survey (not specific to public health) found that 56% of employees cite pay as a top reason to look for a new job, with 41% responding that they would leave for a 5% pay increase.[12] While several studies compare salaries between different occupations within HDs or ask PH WINS respondents if they are satisfied with their salary,[13] fewer contrast salaries for the same occupations within government versus the private sector or ask directly about wage competition.

The American Rescue Plan Act's Public Health Infrastructure Grant[14] provides temporary public health workforce funding, but if salary levels are significantly lower in HDs as compared with competitor employers, recruitment may remain a challenge for HDs. One 2022 study found that the wage gap is so large that at least 1 local HD had to give their workforce funding back to the state because they were unable to fill positions.[15]

The Bureau of Labor Statistics (BLS) gathers data on salaries for each of the occupations for which there is a Standard Occupational Classification (SOC)[16] code. SOC categories are used by BLS and other federal agencies to classify, enumerate, and study 867 detailed occupations. In addition, industries (i.e., types of employer organizations) are categorized with North American Industry Classification System (NAICS) codes.[17] The BLS Occupational Employment and Wage Statistics (OEWS) program provides salary estimates for 830 occupations,[18] including by NAICS industry, allowing comparisons of wages for the individuals working in the same occupation but different industries. Unfortunately, OEWS does not report salary details using the detailed NAICS code for Administration of Public Health Programs (923120),[19] but does allow for salary comparisons between local and state government with nongovernment organizations.

Although SOC codes are an imperfect match with certain occupations in HDs,[20] there are new efforts to match public health occupations with SOC codes to improve workforce research. The public health workforce taxonomy established by the University of Michigan[21] lists 73 occupations in the governmental public health workforce. These occupations, occasionally with slightly different nomenclature, are also used in PH WINS[22] for respondents' "job category." Two recent studies matched these occupations with SOC codes.[8,23]

Using the public health workforce taxonomy, as matched to SOC codes, as well as OEWS data, we asked whether there are salary differences between workers within key occupations in local or state government as compared with workers in the same occupations in other industries.

METHODS

We first used existing workforce taxonomies that matched public health occupations with SOC codes to identify SOC codes to prioritize and analyze, then we analyzed BLS salary data.

Taxonomy Matching and Inclusion/Exclusion Criteria

In a 2023 study, researchers matched the job titles of 26 516 PH WINS 2021 responders using the National Institute for Occupational Safety and Health Industry and Occupation Computerized Coding System.[23] They also referenced a study matching the University of Michigan public health workforce taxonomy with SOC codes, which also used machine learning to match 38 533 public health job postings to SOC codes.[8] After generating a list of the key SOC codes for occupations in HDs, we prioritized occupations requiring specific training or credentialling (i.e., minimum of 1 to 2 years of training or an associate's degree), that are relatively specific to HDs, and that constituted more than 0.5% of PH WINS responses or otherwise are a high priority in the HDs.

Occupations requiring relatively little preparation, such as custodians or administrative assistants, or that serve business support functions across many government agencies, such as accountants, customer service specialists, or human resources professionals, were excluded. We included certain PH WINS job categories known to have a poor SOC match such as disease intervention specialist, grants or contracts specialist, and population health specialist, but indicated the poor match, and excluded categories with no match such as implementation specialist and peer counselor. In addition, several PH WINS job categories matched to the same SOC code (e.g., deputy director, program manager, public health agency director); we selected the most-frequently matched SOC codes that could represent several HD job titles in this situation. We selected 44 SOC codes in all (Table 1 and Appendix A, available as a supplement to the online version of this article at https://ajph.org).

Salary Data Analysis

The OEWS program is a semiannual mail survey of nonfarm establishments and produces employment and wage estimates annually for approximately 830 SOCs, gathering data from every metropolitan and nonmetropolitan area in every state, across all surveyed industries, and from establishments of varying sizes. We used the May 2022 OEWS data, the most recent available.

OEWS also gathers data by industry (using NAICS codes). Although OEWS provides information on salary by occupation for 455 different industries including highly specific industries such as "Theater Companies and Dinner Theaters" (711110), the NAICS-based research "does not generally include government-owned establishments, even when their primary activity would be classified in industries covered by the economic census."[24] A NAICS code for "Administration of Public Health

TABLE 1— Standard Occupational Classification (SOC) Codes Included in Public Health Workforce Salary Analysis, With Code Used in Occupational Employment and Wage Survey (OEWS) if Different, and Estimated Job Category From the Public Health Workforce Interests and Needs Survey (PH WINS)

Standard Occupational Classification (SOC) Title	SOC Code (OEWS SOC if Different)[a]	PH WINS 2021 Job Category/Categories (Estimated)[b]
Chief Executives	11-1011	Department/Bureau Director
General and Operations Managers	11-1021	Department/Bureau Director; Program Director; Deputy Director; Public Health Agency Director; Quality Improvement Worker
Computer and Information Systems Managers	11-3021	Information Systems Manager/Information Technology Specialist
Medical and Health Services Managers	11-9111	Program Director; Department/Bureau Director; Public Health Program Manager; Deputy Director; Public Health Agency Director; Public Health Manager or Program Manager
Social and Community Services Managers	11-9151	Public Health Manager or Program Manager
Emergency Management Directors	11-9161	Emergency Preparedness/Management Worker
Managers, All Other	11-9199	Program Director; Department/Bureau Director; Deputy Director; Emergency Preparedness/Management Worker; Health Officer; Program Evaluator; Public Health Agency Director; Public Health Manager or Program Manager; Quality Improvement Worker; Grants or Contracts Specialist (poor match)
Compliance Officers	13-1041	Licensure/Regulation/Enforcement Worker
Management Analysts	13-1111	Program Evaluator
Computer & Information Research Scientists	15-1221	Public Health Informatics Specialist
Database Administrators	15-1242	Data or Research Analyst
Computer Occupations, All Other	15-1299	Information Systems Manager/Information Technology Specialist
Operations Research Analysts	15-2031	Policy Analyst; Data or Research Analyst
Environmental Engineers	17-2081	Engineer
Microbiologists	19-1022	Laboratory Scientist/Medical Technologist; Laboratory Technician; Laboratory Quality Control Worker
Epidemiologists	19-1041	Epidemiologist
Medical Scientists, Except Epidemiologists	19-1042	Laboratory Scientist/Medical Technologist
Chemists	19-2031	Laboratory Scientist/Medical Technologist; Laboratory Technician
Environmental Scientists and Specialists, Including Health	19-2041	Sanitarian or Inspector; Environmental Health Worker
Political Scientists	19-3094	Policy Analyst
Social Scientists and Related Workers	19-3099 (19-3000)[a]	Program Evaluator
Environmental Science and Protection Technicians, Including Health	19-4091 (19-4042)[a]	Sanitarian or Inspector; Environmental Health Worker
Social Science Research Assistants	19-4061	Data or Research Analyst
Life, Physical, and Social Science Technicians, All Other (includes Quality Control Analysts)	19-4099	Quality Improvement Worker
Occupational Health and Safety Specialists and Technicians	19-5010	Sanitarian or Inspector
Occupational Health and Safety Specialists	19-5011	Environmental Health Worker; Health Officer
Occupational Health and Safety Technicians	19-5012	Sanitarian or Inspector
Substance Abuse and Behavioral Disorder Counselors	21-1011 (21-1018)[a]	Behavioral Health Professional
Healthcare Social Workers	21-1022	Social Worker/Social Services Professional
Mental Health and Substance Abuse Social Workers	21-1023	Social Worker/Social Services Professional; Behavioral Health Professional
Health Education Specialists	21-1091	Health Educator; Health Navigator; Population Health Specialist (poor match)

Continued

TABLE 1— Continued

Standard Occupational Classification (SOC) Title	SOC Code (OEWS SOC if Different)[a]	PH WINS 2021 Job Category/Categories (Estimated)[b]
Social and Human Service Assistants	21-1093	Social Worker/Social Services Professional; Community Health Worker
Community Health Workers	21-1094	Community Health Worker; Disease Intervention Specialist (poor match)
Public Relations Specialists	27-3031	Public Information Specialist
Dietitians and Nutritionists	29-1031	Nutritionist or Dietitian
Registered Nurses	29-1141	Registered Nurse - Public Health or Community Health Nurse; Other Nurse - Clinical Services; Registered Nurse - Unspecified
Nurse Practitioners	29-1171	Nurse Practitioner
Physicians, All Other (including Preventive Medicine Physicians)	29-1229	Public Health/Preventive Medicine Physician
Dental Hygienists	29-1292	Other Oral Health Professional
Clinical Laboratory Technologists and Technicians	29-2012 (29-2010)[a]	Laboratory Technician
Medical Records Specialists	29-2072	Medical/Vital Records Staff
Nursing Assistants	31-1131	Nursing and Home Health Aide
Dental Assistants	31-9091	Other Oral Health Professional
Statistical Assistants	43-9111	Data or Research Analyst

[a]The OEWS from the US Department of Labor occasionally uses slightly different SOC code numbers for occupation titles that are matched to other SOC numbers in other settings. When the SOC codes are different in the usual use of SOC as compared with the code number in OEWS, both numbers are listed.
[b]The "job categories" in PH WINS did not always match clearly with a specific SOC code, and in some cases the same PH WINS job category matched with more than 1 SOC code or vice versa. For certain occupations, the SOC match was especially uncertain; these cases are listed as "poor match."

Programs" exists (923120), but the OEWS data do not use this code. The NAICS codes most relevant to HDs include "State Government, excluding schools and hospitals" (999200), and "Local Government, excluding schools and hospitals" (999300). We compared median salaries in these 2 sectors with salaries in the private or nongovernment sector (defined, in this article, as all other sectors except for government, thus including both for-profit and nonprofit organizations). Because the data are reported in aggregate, statistical analysis of the salary data was not possible. We therefore used descriptive statistics.

RESULTS

Salaries were at least 5% lower in state government than the private sector for 31 occupations, and at least 5% higher for 10 occupations. In local government, salaries were at least 5% lower than private sector for 20 occupations and at least 5% higher for 10 occupations. For 1 occupation, salaries were at least 5% higher in state government than private industry, but lower for local government, and for 2 occupations the opposite was true (Table 2).

Occupations with the severest salary disparities, with median annual salaries paying between 20% and up to 47% lower in either local or state government as compared with the private sector, included management, leadership, program management, program evaluation, and policy occupations. The largest salary disparities were for management occupations including "Chief Executives" (paying up to 46.9% less in government), "Operations Research Analysts" (−35.6%), "Emergency Management Directors" (−33.4%); "Managers, All Other" (−32.6%), "Computer and Information System Managers" (−29.1%), and "Management Analysts" (−26.8%); computer and mathematics occupations including "Computer and Information Research Scientists" (−45.5%) and "Computer Occupations, All Other" (−29.2%); scientific, technical, and research occupations including "Political Scientists" (the SOC code for "Policy Analysts," −33.5%), "Epidemiologists" (−25%), and "Chemists" (i.e., laboratory scientists, −21.4%); and 1 clinical occupation, "Dental Hygienists" (−23.8%).

Other inspection or compliance roles, scientific roles, technicians, and clinicians had moderate disparities in salary (paying 10%–19% less in either state or local government), including

TABLE 2— Salary Difference for Public Health Occupations From Occupational Employment and Wage Survey (OEWS) Median Annual Salaries, Private Sector Versus Local or State Government

SOC Title	SOC Code	Private Sector/ Nongovernment Median Annual Salary, $	Local Government, Excluding Schools and Hospitals, Median Annual Salary, $	State Government, Excluding Schools and Hospitals, Median Annual Salary, $	Salary Difference: Local Government/ Private Sector, $	Salary Difference: State Government/ Private Sector, $	% Decrease/ Increase: Local/ Private	% Decrease/ Increase: State/ Private
Chief Executives[a]	11-1011	209 810	111 380	129 540	−98 430	−80 270	−46.91	−38.26
General and Operations Managers[b]	11-1021	97 030	105 860	103 550	8 830	6 520	9.10	6.72
Computer and Information Systems Managers[a]	11-3021	166 070	126 930	117 690	−39 140	−48 380	−23.57	−29.13
Medical and Health Services Managers[a]	11-9111	103 940	103 510	94 640	−430	−9 300	−0.41	−8.95
Social and Community Service Managers[b]	11-9151	69 260	96 070	80 040	26 810	10 780	38.71	15.56
Emergency Management Directors[a]	11-9161	100 210	75 160	66 750	−25 050	−33 460	−25.00	−33.39
Managers, All Other[a]	11-9199	130 330	103 580	87 820	−26 750	−42 510	−20.52	−32.62
Compliance Officers[a]	13-1041	69 990	64 000	59 700	−5 990	−10 290	−8.56	−14.70
Management Analysts[a]	13-1111	98 500	83 180	72 090	−15 320	−26 410	−15.55	−26.81
Computer and Information Research Scientists[a]	15-1221	156 620	85 360	NA	−71 260	NA	−45.50	
Database Administrators[a]	15-1242	102 240	99 820	84 470	−2 420	−17 770	−2.37	−17.38
Computer Occupations, All Other[a]	15-1299	96 440	68 290	75 190	−28 150	−21 250	−29.19	−22.03
Operations Research Analysts[a]	15-2031	86 430	83 930	55 650	−2 500	−30 780	−2.89	−35.61
Environmental Engineers[a]	17-2081	96 320	95 370	87 710	−950	−8 610	−0.99	−8.94
Microbiologists[c]	19-1022	80 890	83 440	63 500	2 550	−17 390	3.15	−21.50
Epidemiologists[a]	19-1041	92 700	70 910	69 510	−21 790	−23 190	−23.51	−25.02
Medical Scientists, Except Epidemiologists[a]	19-1042	102 210	86 770	86 300	−15 440	−15 910	−15.11	−15.57
Chemists[a]	19-2031	80 010	76 640	62 930	−3 370	−17 080	−4.21	−21.35
Environmental Scientists and Specialists, Including Health[a]	19-2041	76 870	76 300	70 080	−570	−6 790	−0.74	−8.83
Social Scientists and Related Workers[a]	19-3000	83 210	79 290	80 450	−3 920	−2 760	−4.71	−3.32
Political Scientists[a]	19-3094	103 730	86 960	68 950	−16 770	−34 780	−16.17	−33.53
Environmental Science and Protection Technicians, Including Health[b]	19-4042	46 710	58 710	50 590	12 000	3 880	25.69	8.31
Social Science Research Assistants[a]	19-4061	51 490	48 960	41 540	−2 530	−9950	−4.91	−19.32
	19-4099	50 080	60 870	38 750	10 790	−11 330	21.55	−22.62

Continued

AJPH March 2024, Vol. 114, No. 3

TABLE 2— Continued

SOC Title	SOC Code	Private Sector/ Nongovernment Median Annual Salary, $	Local Government, Excluding Schools and Hospitals, Median Annual Salary, $	State Government, Excluding Schools and Hospitals, Median Annual Salary, $	Salary Difference: Local Government/ Private Sector, $	Salary Difference: State Government/ Private Sector, $	% Decrease/ Increase: Local/ Private	% Decrease/ Increase: State/ Private
Life, Physical, and Social Science Technicians, All Other[c]								
Occupational Health and Safety Specialists and Technicians[a]	19-5010	75 050	67 720	64 310	−7 330	−10 740	−9.77	−14.31
Occupational Health and Safety Specialists[a]	19-5011	78 650	73 030	65 150	−5 620	−13 500	−7.15	−17.16
Occupational Health and Safety Technicians[c]	19-5012	58 240	61 450	53 850	3 210	−4 390	5.51	−7.54
Substance Abuse, Behavioral Disorder, and Mental Health Counselors[b]	21-1018	48 820	62 050	51 110	13 230	2 290	27.10	4.69
Healthcare Social Workers[a]	21-1022	60 370	54 930	51 400	−5 440	−8 970	−9.01	−14.86
Mental Health and Substance Abuse Social Workers[b]	21-1023	49 170	61 280	60 250	12 110	11 080	24.63	22.53
Health Education Specialists[a]	21-1091	58 860	55 490	55 190	−3 370	−3 670	−5.73	−6.24
Social and Human Service Assistants[b]	21-1093	37 630	46 790	41 520	9 160	3 890	24.34	10.34
Community Health Workers[b]	21-1094	45 570	47 770	47 840	2 200	2 270	4.83	4.98
Public Relations Specialists[c]	27-3031	67 160	69 270	62 940	2 110	−4 220	3.14	−6.28
Dietitians and Nutritionists[a]	29-1031	66 630	60 320	57 450	−6 310	−9 180	−9.47	−13.78
Registered Nurses[a]	29-1141	80 970	79 590	77 610	−1 380	−3 360	−1.70	−4.15
Nurse Practitioners[a]	29-1171	121 520	116 900	102 820	−4 620	−18 700	−3.80	−15.39
Physicians, All Other[a]	29-1229	217 150	210 370	175 800	−6 780	−41 350	−3.12	−19.04
Dental Hygienists[a]	29-1292	81 470	78 240	62 110	−3 230	−19 360	−3.96	−23.76
Clinical Laboratory Technologists and Technicians[a]	29-2010	56 820	51 810	48 110	−5 010	−8 710	−8.82	−15.33
Medical Records Specialists[c]	29-2072	46 770	44 370	49 650	−2 400	2 880	−5.13	6.16
Nursing Assistants[b]	31-1131	35 640	37 400	37 330	1 760	1 690	4.94	4.74
Dental Assistants[c]	31-9091	44 820	44 510	50 960	−310	6 140	−0.69	13.70
Statistical Assistants[c]	43-9111	51 830	53 020	44 530	1 190	−7 300	2.30	−14.08

Note. NA = no data available; SOC = Standard Occupational Classification.
[a]Pays less in government than private sector.
[b]Pays more in government than private sector.
[c]Higher salaries in state government than private sector and lower in local government than private sector, or vice versa.

"Compliance Officers," "Database Administrators," "Medical Scientists, Except Epidemiologists," "Social Science Research Assistants," "Occupational Health and Safety Specialists," "Healthcare Social Workers," "Dieticians and Nutritionists," "Nurse Practitioners," "Physicians, All Other," "Clinical Laboratory Technologists and Technicians," and "Statistical Assistants."

Some occupations had higher salaries in local and state government than in private industry. Those with the largest wage advantage in government were primarily in "Community and Social Service Occupations" or related human services roles, including "Social and Community Service Managers," earning up to 38.7% more in government, as well as "Substance Use Counselors" (+27%) and "Mental Health Social Workers" (+24.6%). Certain technician roles paid more in government, such as "Environmental Science and Protection Technician" (+25.7%) and "Social Services Assistants" (+24.3%).

The BLS data show only a small wage gap for registered nurses (RNs), conflicting with other research showing a much larger disparity.[7] Because there is no separate SOC code for public health nurses (PHNs), they are mixed in with RNs.[23] It is possible that RNs working in carceral facilities, state-funded long-term-care facilities, human services, or other government agencies besides HDs earn more than PHNs, skewing the median salaries higher than it would be if it pertained exclusively to PHNs.

We also assessed the proportion of workers in each occupation working in different NAICS industry groups to determine if wage differences might be explained by competition from certain industries (Appendix B, C, and D, available as supplements to the online version of this article at https://ajph.org).

According to OEWS, "Professional, Scientific, and Technical Services" (Sector 54), which includes consulting firms and research services, hired between 10% and 50% of several occupations with wage disparities, such as "Epidemiologists," "Management Analysts," "Social Scientists," "Political Scientists," "Occupational Health & Safety Specialists," "Compliance Officers," "Computer & Information Research Scientists," "Computer and Information Systems Managers," "Environmental Scientists and Specialists, Including Health," and "Environmental Engineers." "Health Care and Social Assistance" employed large numbers of "Epidemiologists," "Social Scientists," "Dietitians and Nutritionists," "Compliance Officers," "Dental Hygienists," and "Emergency Management Directors." "Manufacturing" and "Construction" hired large numbers of "Occupational Health & Safety Specialists," and "Finance and Insurance" is a major employer of "Compliance Officers" and "Computer and Information Systems Managers." The "Information" sector is a key employer of computer occupations.

For the occupations that pay more in government, competitor industries tended to be in "Health Care and Social Assistance" for "Social Services Managers," "Mental Health Social Workers," and "Healthcare Social Workers." Looking in more detail at the "Health Care and Social Assistance" sector (NAICS 62), however, the subsectors within NAICS 62 that hire occupations that pay more in government tend to be substance abuse centers, nursing and residential care facilities, and social assistance (nonprofit) organizations, as opposed to large health care providers or hospitals. This is especially the case for "helping" professions such as social work or counseling. The top detailed NAICS Health Care and Social Assistance subsectors for occupations paying less in government include "Hospitals" hiring "Epidemiologists," "Dietitians and Nutritionists," and "Emergency Management Directors" and "Offices of Dentists" hiring "Dental Hygienists." By contrast, the top detailed NAICS health care and social assistance subsectors for occupations paying more in government included "Ambulatory Health Care Services" and "Outpatient Mental Health and Substance Abuse Centers" hiring "Mental Health Social Workers" and "Nursing and Residential Care Facilities" and "Social Assistance" hiring "Social & Community Services Managers."

DISCUSSION

Salary differences for many, but not all, occupations appear substantial, especially for technical, research, management, and leadership roles. Based on the limited federal data available, many public health occupations in local or state government appear to face serious wage competition, especially from the for-profit sector, particularly from professional, scientific, and technical services; finance and insurance; and information sectors, and from large health care organizations.

HDs have faced a decades-long workforce shortage.[1,2] While more research is needed to identify the impact of wage differences, it seems that the fact that between 20 and 31 of the identified occupations in this study pay at least 5% less in government—a differential that has been shown to entice workers to quit[12]—may have contributed to this shortage. Close attention should to be paid to whether the historic Public Health Infrastructure Grant investment, which recommended HDs to pay fair salaries to grant-funded hires, might result in long-term wage increases for permanent workers.[14] And though more public health students might be graduating, labor market mismatches can still cause workforce shortages.[25–29]

Wages and funding in the public sector are often set by factors unrelated to competition in the job market, including civil service pay scales, union-negotiated pay scales, local or state regulations, and the choices of elected officials.

Private-sector employers are not typically bound by these restrictions and can respond to a workforce shortage by increasing salaries, improving benefits, providing sign-on bonuses, and purchasing recruitment advertising or services. Within the private sector, for-profit corporations in particular generally have more revenue to invest in such efforts. SOC occupations with higher numbers of workers in industries comprising for-profit corporations, such as computer programmers, engineers, and scientists, may experience more labor market competition.[8,25,26] Meanwhile, occupations in which large numbers of workers are employed by small nonprofit organizations, such as social workers, may earn more in government. For certain technician occupations ("Environmental Science and Protection Technician" and "Social Services Assistants"), which require less credentialling and pay more in government, union-negotiated pay scales may cause government salaries to be higher.

Considering the potential recruitment challenges caused by salary disparities for certain occupations, several policy solutions might be considered.

Improvements in Federal Data

To improve federal data on the public health workforce, including for clearer salary information and workforce enumeration, BLS should be encouraged to use more detailed NAICS codes for OEWS if possible, including consistently using the specific NAICS code for public health services when surveying local and state governments,[23] and establish more-specific SOC codes for certain occupations like PHNs.[30,31]

Improving Salaries

For those occupations with higher salaries in HDs, higher wages should be emphasized in recruitment marketing campaigns, whereas for those paying less, salary increases should be considered. Benchmarking salaries with competitor sectors is a standard procedure in human resources. It is also crucial for diversity and inclusion.[32–34] However, changing salary grades in government can be difficult, especially in jurisdictions where there are complex regulations, collective bargaining agreements, or political factors that make salary increases for government workers difficult.[11,35–37] State and local government wages have stagnated over the last 15 years.[38] Increasing salaries to recruit new hires can also cause wage compression with longer-serving or senior staff, or between union and nonunion employees, and, if budgets are stagnant, increasing wages for current staff means fewer new openings are available. Advocacy efforts at local, state, and federal levels would be needed to increase funding, improve HD salaries, and fill workforce gaps.[37] Because there are approximately 3000 local and state HDs, each with its own hiring regulations—some with civil service hiring laws embedded in their state constitutions—regulatory reforms to improve public-sector salaries are likely a long-term challenge.

If wage increases are possible, HDs could use local wage benchmarking and analysis of "hard-to-fill" vacancies to prioritize mission-critical occupations with large wage gaps for salary increases.

Recruitment Strategies in Absence of Higher Wages

Strategy 1: Benefits. If salaries cannot be increased in the short term, HDs may consider other strategies to attract candidates. While salary is crucial, job seekers also consider benefits, work–life balance, schedule, and public service motivation. A survey of public health students found that "Job security (84.7%), competitive benefits (82.2%), identifying with the mission of the organization (82.2%), and opportunities for training/continuing education (80.6%)" were key motivators to work for government, though competitive salary was a detractor.[39]

Even if salary is lower, government agencies often have certain advantages for job seekers that could serve as recruitment incentives if they are well-marketed to job seekers. Government may offer better retirement plans, with 86% of state and local government workers having access to defined benefit retirement plans (pensions), compared with 15% of private-sector workers, and with 68% of government staff receiving health care coverage compared with 47% in private sector.[40]

In one study, employees who came to HDs from private industry were attracted by benefits and job security.[41] The 2022 Global Benefits Attitudes survey found that 59% of respondents were willing to trade lower compensation for more generous retirement benefits and 46% for better health care plans.[12] However, the same survey found that 56% of employees cite pay as a top reason to look for a new job; only 29% listed retirement benefits as a reason to leave.

Using strong retirement benefits may not help as much with recruiting younger staff.[42] When asked what they most want employers to focus on, individuals born from 1950 to 1980 mentioned retirement, but workers born 1981 or after listed other priorities.[13]

Some government agencies also provide overtime pay, which is not generally well-advertised to potential hires. Union membership is more than 5 times higher in government than the private sector, and the advantages of union protection can be marketed to job seekers.[43] Government agencies sometimes have better work–life balance and more provide wellness benefits.[40] However, some data show that the value of benefits in government employers has declined over the years and that compensation lags behind the private sector even when including the value of benefits.[38]

Strategy 2: Public service motivation. Many job seekers are motivated by the desire for meaningful work or public service. One study showed that participants were willing to be paid $17 300 to $22 639 less in average annual income to work in a more meaningful job.[44] However, careers in nonprofit organizations and other sectors are also highly meaningful, and relying on workers to take lower salaries in exchange for meaningful work, while noble in spirit, is neither equitable nor sustainable. With harassment caused by COVID-19, worker motivation to serve the public could be reduced.[45]

Strategy 3: Recruitment marketing and onboarding. There are new efforts to improve the image of public health and attract job applicants to HDs,[46–51] and new initiatives to improve onboarding and employee wellness and to change structures that cause burnout may improve retention.[52–54]

Strategy 4: Student loan repayment. For professions for which advanced education is required, student loan debt could force some job candidates to choose higher-paying jobs in other sectors.[55] Federal data show that for Master of Public Health graduates, median postgraduate earnings were $48 866, but loan debt was $52 263.[44] Considering the racial disparities in student loan debt,[56] comparably low salaries could create challenges for recruitment and retention of diverse candidates.

The Public Health Workforce Loan Repayment program, approved in the 2022 Omnibus Bill,[57] would provide student loan repayment for individuals with graduate degrees in public health, laboratory sciences, informatics, or statistics who choose to work in HDs for a period of 3 years. If funded, it could provide an incentive to candidates to work in HDs.

Limitations

Because BLS does not use the NAICS code for public health, for certain occupations, especially broad-based occupations like "senior executives," there is a high chance that the majority of BLS data regarding local or state government is not specifically representative of HDs. Wages and costs of living are very different in different parts of the country, but geographic analysis was beyond the scope of this study.[58] Some HDs allow fully remote work, while others prohibit it. Further research is needed to assess the impact of remote work options—for example, to assess whether HDs that require in-person work, especially in locations with higher costs of living, might face compounded challenges from lower wages.

Because "public health nurse" is not a separate SOC code, it is hard to know which of the salaries pertain to a health care environment as opposed to public health. This may also be the case for social workers or counselors because there are likely to be more behavioral health staff working for human services agencies, as opposed to HDs. This is less likely to be the case for epidemiologists or health educators, who are more likely to work in HDs.

Certain jobs in a local or state government agency might require different responsibilities than in other sectors, which might result in different pay; further research such as an analysis of job postings may clarify this potential difference.

While benefits are often better in government than private industry, we did not include the cash value of benefits in this analysis.[38] Future research using PH WINS data to assess any links between respondents expressing a desire to quit and working in a comparably lower-paying occupation could clarify the impact of lower wages on retention.

Public Health Implications

If computer professionals earn up to $48 380 more outside government, we may ask who will implement new initiatives to modernize public health data infrastructure.[14] When epidemiologists can earn $23 000 more and emergency management directors $33 460 more by quitting their jobs in HDs to work in private industry, we might wonder who will respond to the next pandemic or public health emergency. And with hundreds of senior HD leaders having quit, retired, or been fired during the pandemic,[2,45] we may ask how new leadership will be recruited when chief executives can nearly double their salaries and earn $98 430 more outside government.

Improving recruitment marketing, including focusing on benefits and meaningful work, combined with improved salaries or loan repayment, may help bolster the workforce, but stagnant funding and salaries will remain a barrier to public health.

Conclusions

To sustainably recruit and retain the diverse workforce that is needed to keep our nation healthy, we must consider salary disparities in health departments as an upstream determinant of public health. AJPH

ABOUT THE AUTHORS

Heather Krasna, Malvika Venkataraman, and Isabella Patino are with Columbia University Mailman School of Public Health, New York, NY.

CORRESPONDENCE

Correspondence should be sent to Heather Krasna, 722 W 168 St, New York, NY 10032 (e-mail: hk2778@cumc.columbia.edu). Reprints can be ordered at https://ajph.org by clicking the "Reprints" link.

PUBLICATION INFORMATION

Full Citation: Krasna H, Venkataraman M, Patino I. Salary disparities in public health occupations: analysis of federal data, 2021–2022. *Am J Public Health*. 2024;114(3):329–339.

Acceptance Date: October 21, 2023.

DOI: https://doi.org/10.2105/AJPH.2023.307512

ORCID iDs:

Heather Krasna https://orcid.org/0000-0002-4820-9773

CONTRIBUTORS

H. Krasna conceptualized and wrote the article. M. Venkataraman and I. Patino coded data and conducted analysis.

ACKNOWLEDGMENTS

This project was supported by Centers for Disease Control and Prevention and Health Resources and Services Administration under awards U81HP47167 and UR2HP47371. This article is dedicated to all public health workers who deserve a raise.

CONFLICTS OF INTEREST

The authors have no conflicts of interest to disclose.

HUMAN PARTICIPANT PROTECTION

The study was considered not human subjects research under 45 CFR 46 by Columbia University's institutional review board (IRB-AAAU3962).

REFERENCES

1. Draper DA, Hurley RE, Lauer J. Public health workforce shortages imperil nation's health. *Res Brief.* 2008;(4):1–8.
2. Leider JP, Castrucci BC, Robins M, et al. The exodus of state and local public health employees: separations started before and continued throughout COVID-19. *Health Aff (Millwood).* 2023;42(3):338–348. https://doi.org/10.1377/hlthaff.2022.01251
3. Beck AJ, Boulton ML, Lemmings J, Clayton JL. Challenges to recruitment and retention of the state health department epidemiology workforce. *Am J Prev Med*. 2012;42(1):76–80. https://doi.org/10.1016/j.amepre.2011.08.021
4. Boulton ML, Hadler J, Beck AJ, Ferland L, Lichtveld M. Assessment of epidemiology capacity in state health departments, 2004–2009. *Public Health Rep*. 2011;126(1):84–93. https://doi.org/10.1177/003335491112600112
5. Beck AJ, Boulton ML. The public health nurse workforce in US state and local health departments, 2012. *Public Health Rep*. 2016;131(1):145–152. https://doi.org/10.1177/003335491613100121
6. Yeager VA, Wisniewski JM. Factors that influence the recruitment and retention of nurses in public health agencies. *Public Health Rep*. 2017;132(5):556–562. https://doi.org/10.1177/0033354917719704
7. Issel LM, Lurie CF, Bekemeier B. Wage inequity: within-market comparative analysis of salary for public health nurses and hospital nurses. *J Public Health Manag Pract*. 2016;22(6):550–558. https://doi.org/10.1097/PHH.0000000000000390
8. Krasna H, Czabanowska K, Beck A, Cushman LF, Leider JP. Labour market competition for public health graduates in the United States: a comparison of workforce taxonomies with job postings before and during the COVID-19 pandemic. *Int J Health Plann Manage*. 2021;36(suppl 1):151–167. https://doi.org/10.1002/hpm.3128
9. Perry JL. Bringing society in: toward a theory of public-service motivation. *J Public Adm Res Theory*. 2000;10(2):471–488. https://doi.org/10.1093/oxfordjournals.jpart.a024277
10. Yeager VA, Leider JP. The role of salary in recruiting employees in state and local governmental public health: PH WINS 2017. *Am J Public Health*. 2019;109(5):683–685. https://doi.org/10.2105/AJPH.2019.305008
11. Michaels I, Pirani S, Fleming M, et al. Enumeration of the public health workforce in New York State: workforce changes in the wake of COVID-19. *Int J Environ Res Public Health*. 2022;19(20):13592. https://doi.org/10.3390/ijerph192013592
12. WTW. 2022 Global Benefits Attitudes Survey. Available at: https://www.wtwco.com/en-us/form-thank-you/2022/11/hwc-hb-usa-usa-wgc-20221111-global-benefits-attitudes-pg10421a1-03-lp-gated-confirmation. Accessed June 12, 2023.
13. Sellers K, Leider JP, Gould E, et al. The state of the US governmental public health workforce, 2014–2017. *Am J Public Health*. 2019;109(5):674–680. https://doi.org/10.2105/AJPH.2019.305011
14. Centers for Disease Control and Prevention. Public Health Infrastructure Grant Program. August 9, 2023. Available at: https://www.cdc.gov/infrastructure/index.html. Accessed October 6, 2023.
15. Kirkland C, Oldfield-Tabbert K, Karnik H, Orr J, Martin S, Leider JP. Public health workforce gaps, impacts, and improvement strategies from COVID-19. *Int J Environ Res Public Health*. 2022;19(20):13084. https://doi.org/10.3390/ijerph192013084
16. US Bureau of Labor Statistics. Standard Occupational Classification. Available at: https://www.bls.gov/soc. Accessed December 22, 2019.
17. US Census Bureau. North American Industry Classification System. Available at: https://www.census.gov/naics. Accessed April 16, 2023.
18. US Bureau of Labor Statistics. Occupational employment and wage statistics. Available at: https://www.bls.gov/oes. Accessed October 7, 2023.
19. NAICS Association. NAICS code description. 923120 Administration of public health programs. Available at: https://www.naics.com/naics-code-description/?code=923120. Accessed April 16, 2023.
20. American Public Health Association. Advancing efforts to enumerate and characterize the nation's public health workforce. November 5, 2013. Available at: https://www.apha.org/policies-and-advocacy/public-health-policy-statements/policy-database/2014/07/08/07/50/advancing-efforts-to-enumerate-and-characterize-the-nations-public-health-workforce. Accessed April 6, 2023.
21. Boulton ML, Beck AJ, Coronado F, et al. Public health workforce taxonomy. *Am J Prev Med*. 2014;47(5, suppl 3):S314–S323. https://doi.org/10.1016/j.amepre.2014.07.015
22. Sellers K, Leider J, Harper E, et al. The Public Health Workforce Interests and Needs Survey: the first national survey of state health agency employees. *J Public Health Manag Pract*. 2015;21(suppl 6):S13–S27. https://doi.org/10.1097/PHH.0000000000000331
23. Krasna H, Venkataraman M, Robins M, Patino I, Leider J. Standard Occupational Classification

codes: gaps in federal data on the public health workforce. *Am J Public Health*. 2024;114(1):48–56. https://doi.org/10.2105/AJPH.2023.307463

24. US Census Bureau. Economic census: NAICS codes & understanding industry classification systems. Available at: https://www.census.gov/programs-surveys/economic-census/year/2022/guidance/understanding-naics.html. Accessed May 2, 2023.
25. Vujicic M, Zurn P. The dynamics of the health labour market. *Int J Health Plann Manage*. 2006;21(2):101–115. https://doi.org/10.1002/hpm.834
26. Krasna H. Public Health Graduates in the United States: Employment Outcomes and Employer Demand. Doctoral thesis. Maastricht University; 2021. Available at: https://cris.maastrichtuniversity.nl/en/publications/public-health-graduates-in-the-united-states-employment-outcomes-. Accessed October 7, 2023.
27. Krasna H, Kornfeld J, Cushman L, Ni S, Antoniou P, March D. The new public health workforce: employment outcomes of public health graduate students. *J Public Health Manag Pract*. 2019;27(1):12–19. https://doi.org/10.1097/PHH.0000000000000976
28. Erwin PC, Beck AJ, Yeager VA, Leider JP. Public health undergraduates in the workforce: a trickle, soon a wave? *Am J Public Health*. 2019;109(5):685–687. https://doi.org/10.2105/AJPH.2019.305004
29. Leider JP, Plepys CM, Castrucci BC, Burke EM, Blakely CH. Trends in the conferral of graduate public health degrees: a triangulated approach. *Public Health Rep*. 2018;133(6):729–737. https://doi.org/10.1177/0033354918791542
30. Gebbie K, Merrill J, Sanders L, Gebbie EN, Chen DW. Public health workforce enumeration: beware the "quick fix." *J Public Health Manag Pract*. 2007;13(1):72–79. https://doi.org/10.1097/00124784-200701000-00012
31. Gebbie KM. *The Public Health Work Force: Enumeration 2000*. US Department of Health and Human Services, Health Resources and Services Administration, Bureau of Health Professions, National Center for Health Workforce Information and Analysis; 2000. Available at: https://www.google.com/books/edition/The_Public_Health_Work_Force/IKW6K0knM4cC?hl=en&gbpv=1&printsec= frontcover. Accessed January 16, 2024.
32. Coronado F, Beck AJ, Shah G, Young JL, Sellers K, Leider JP. Understanding the dynamics of diversity in the public health workforce. *J Public Health Manag Pract*. 2020;26(4):389–392. https://doi.org/10.1097/PHH.0000000000001075
33. Bouye KE, McCleary KJ, Williams KB. Increasing diversity in the health professions: reflections on student pipeline programs. *J Healthc Sci Humanit*. 2016;6(1):67–79.
34. Kapadia F. Health equity requires public health workforce diversity and inclusivity: a public health of consequence, September 2023. *Am J Public Health*. 2023;113(9):936–938. https://doi.org/10.2105/AJPH.2023.307372
35. Sparer MS, Brown LD. Politics and the public health workforce: lessons suggested from a five-state study. *Milbank Q*. 2023;101(3):815–840. https://doi.org/10.1111/1468-0009.12657
36. Barrett K, Greene R. Can government hiring get out of the Stone Age? *Governing*. January 29, 2016. Available at: https://www.governing.com/topics/mgmt/gov-government-hiring-best-practices.html. Accessed November 24, 2020.
37. Ravenhall S. Advocating for a robust public health workforce. *J Public Health Manag Pract*. 2023;29(1):112–113. https://doi.org/10.1097/PHH.0000000000001682
38. Heywood J, Bender K. Out of balance? Comparing public and private sector compensation over 20 years. National Institute on Retirement Security. April 2010. Available at: https://www.nirsonline.org/reports/out-of-balance-comparing-public-and-private-sector-compensation-over-20-years. Accessed June 12, 2023.
39. Yeager VA, Beitsch LM, Johnson SM, Halverson PK. Public health graduates and employment in governmental public health: factors that facilitate and deter working in this setting. *J Public Health Manag Pract*. 2019;27(1):4–11. https://doi.org/10.1097/PHH.0000000000001052
40. US Bureau of Labor Statistics. EBS latest numbers. Available at: https://www.bls.gov/ebs/latest-numbers.htm. Accessed June 11, 2023.
41. Yeager VA, Wisniewski JM, Amos K, Bialek R. What matters in recruiting public health employees: considerations for filling workforce gaps. *Am J Public Health*. 2015;105(12):e33–e36. https://doi.org/10.2105/AJPH.2015.302805
42. WTW. Infographic: Half of US employees face retirement risks. July 11, 2022. Available at: https://www.wtwco.com/en-us/insights/2022/07/infographic-half-of-us-employees-face-retirement-risks. Accessed June 11, 2023.
43. US Bureau of Labor Statistics. Union members summary. January 19, 2023. Available at: https://www.bls.gov/news.release/union2.nr0.htm. Accessed June 11, 2023.
44. Beck AJ, Leider JP, Krasna H, Resnick BA. Monetary and nonmonetary costs and benefits of a public health master's degree in the 21st century. *Am J Public Health*. 2020;110(7):978–985. https://doi.org/10.2105/AJPH.2020.305648
45. Fraser MR. Harassment of health officials: a significant threat to the public's health. *Am J Public Health*. 2022;112(5):728–730. https://doi.org/10.2105/AJPH.2022.306797
46. Seltzer B, Krasna H. *101+ Careers in Public Health*. 3rd ed. New York, NY: Springer Publishing Company; 2021.
47. Krasna H, Kulik PG, Karnik H, Leider JP. Recruiting new talent for public health jobs with evidence-based job descriptions and attractive job postings. *J Public Health Manag Pract*. 2023;29(5):E162–E168. https://doi.org/10.1097/PHH.0000000000001776
48. Krasna H. Region 2 Public Health Training Center. Recruitment toolkit. Available at: https://region2phtc.org/recruitment-toolkit. Accessed October 1, 2022.
49. Public Health Careers.org. Careers in public health. Available at: https://www.publichealthcareers.org. Accessed October 7, 2023.
50. Acheampong NAA. Reward preferences of the youngest generation: attracting, recruiting, and retaining Generation Z into public sector organizations. *Compens Benefits Rev*. 2021;53(2):75–97. https://doi.org/10.1177/0886368720954803
51. Locke R, McGinty M, Guerrero Ramirez G, Sellers K. Attracting new talent to the governmental public health workforce: strategies for improved recruitment of public health graduates. *J Public Health Manag Pract*. 2021;28(1):E235–E243. https://doi.org/10.1097/PHH.0000000000001336
52. Manske J, Hayes H, Zahner S. The new to public health residency program supports transition to public health practice. *J Public Health Manag Pract*. 2022;28(5):E728–E733. https://doi.org/10.1097/PHH.0000000000001569
53. Jackson Preston P. We must practice what we preach: a framework to promote well-being and sustainable performance in the public health workforce in the United States. *J Public Health Policy*. 2022;43(1):140–148. https://doi.org/10.1057/s41271-021-00335-5
54. Schenk KD, Lankau EW, Todd J, Barishansky RM, Nichols GP, Arellano AM. We are the public health workforce. *Health Affairs Forefront*. April 10, 2023. Available at: https://www.healthaffairs.org/content/forefront/we-public-health-workforce. Accessed October 6, 2023.
55. Park C, Coles E. The impact of student debt on career choices among Doctor of Public Health graduates in the United States: a descriptive analysis. *Int J Environ Res Public Health*. 2022;19(8):4836. https://doi.org/10.3390/ijerph19084836
56. Addo FR, Houle JN, Simon D. Young, Black, and (still) in the red: parental wealth, race, and student loan debt. *Race Soc Probl*. 2016;8(1):64–76. https://doi.org/10.1007/s12552-016-9162-0
57. Connolly GE. Consolidated Appropriations Act 2023, HR 2617, 117th Cong (2021–2022). Available at: https://www.congress.gov/bill/117th-congress/house-bill/2617. Accessed May 2, 2023.
58. Sellers K, Leider JP, Bogaert K, Allen JD, Castrucci BC. Making a living in governmental public health: variation in earnings by employee characteristics and work setting. *J Public Health Manag Pract*. 2019;25(suppl 2):S87–S95. https://doi.org/10.1097/PHH.0000000000000935

Health Risks of Unaccompanied Immigrant Children in Federal Custody and in US Communities

Janine Young, MD, Warren Binford, JD, EdM, Michael Garcia Bochenek, JD, and Jordan Greenbaum, MD

Unaccompanied immigrant children continue to arrive at the US–Mexico border and are at high risk for ongoing abuse, neglect, and poor mental and physical health.

We are medical and legal experts in the fields of immigrant and refugee health, child abuse, and the legal rights of international refugee and migrant children. We provide an overview of US federal agencies with custody of unaccompanied immigrant children, a summary of medical care provided while in custody, and recent findings from the independent *Juvenile Care Monitor Report* mandating new custodial conditions for immigrant children while in federal custody.

We provide recommendations to improve the health and well-being of unaccompanied immigrant children while in custody and once released to US sponsors. (*Am J Public Health*. 2024;114(3):340–346. https://doi.org/10.2105/AJPH.2023.307570)

AJPH March 2024, Vol. 114, No. 3

Since 2012, more than 600 000 unaccompanied immigrant children[1] of all ages have immigrated to the United States, with almost 130 000 arriving in fiscal year 2022.[2] A large number of unaccompanied children arrive from the Northern Triangle countries of Central America: Guatemala, El Salvador, and Honduras. Many unaccompanied immigrant children are fleeing poverty, gang violence, abuse, neglect, sexual violence, and natural disasters and experience additional trauma during and after their immigration journey.[3] They are at high risk for physical and mental health issues, including acute injury, malnutrition, dehydration, pregnancy, sexual and physical assault, sexually transmitted infections, posttraumatic stress disorder, and depression.[4] Their unaccompanied immigrant status, young age, social marginalization, and other factors render them at high risk for trafficking and other forms of exploitation both outside and inside the United States.[5–7]

There are 2 federal agencies, the US Department of Homeland Security (DHS) and the US Department of Health and Human Services (HHS), that are the initial legal custodians for unaccompanied immigrant children. We provide a summary of their movement through these 2 federal agencies and medical care provided while in custody, which is based on our extensive experience working with unaccompanied immigrant children as well as findings from the independent *Juvenile Care Monitor Report* issued in January 2023 as a result of a 2022 legal settlement mandating new custodial conditions for immigrant children in federal custody.[8] To our knowledge, this is the only detailed description of the process published by an external source. We provide recommendations to address identified gaps in the care of unaccompanied immigrant children.

CUSTOMS AND BORDER PROTECTION

At the time of apprehension, DHS's Customs and Border Protection (CBP) ordinarily takes custody of unaccompanied immigrant children and should transfer them to HHS's Office of Refugee Resettlement (ORR) custody within 72 hours.[9,10] CBP agents are responsible for initially identifying children who are in acute medical distress after grueling overland travel that may last weeks to months and includes risks of severe dehydration, acute to chronic malnutrition, heat exposure, sexual and physical assault, trauma from border wall falls,[11] and respiratory infections. These conditions may be life threatening in and of themselves, but the risk is exacerbated when children have unidentified comorbid conditions, such as undiagnosed congenital heart malformations, asthma, and severe anemia from chronic poor nutrition. Such diagnoses are easily missed by CBP staff, who have neither training in pediatric medicine nor general medical care, and place children's health at risk.

Once brought to CBP sites—which may take hours or up to several days, during which time these children have no access to any formal medical evaluation, shelter, food, or latrines[12]—initial health interviews are completed by emergency medical technicians, who also lack advanced training in pediatric medicine and can easily miss that infants or children are in medical distress.[8] Within 24 hours of being put in custody, the children receive a limited health screening performed by either a nurse practitioner or a physician assistant (with on-call pediatrician consultation available if medical issues are identified).[8] Medications for acute and chronic issues are provided, and children with identified urgent health needs are referred to local health systems for further evaluation, work-up, and management.[8] Several pediatricians provide on-call support, clinical protocols, and chart reviews to ensure that standards of care are met.[8] Of note, only children in visible distress are provided further mental health services; unaccompanied immigrant children are not formally screened for mental health issues while in CBP custody.[8]

Per the *Juvenile Care Monitor Report*, noted deficiencies in the current model include wide variation in how medical protocols are implemented at CBP sites, including inadequate medical evaluations for older children with chronic medical issues, lack of continuation of chronic medications, absence of repeat health evaluations for children held for longer than 72 hours, and lack of provision of medical information to caregivers or medical providers once children are relinquished to ORR shelters as well as inadequate medical supervision when there are surges in the number of detained children.[8] Also of note are reports of acute medical issues directly related to a chronic condition not being diagnosed and addressed.[8] In such cases, accurate recognition and response may require more extensive clinical pediatric training than nurse practitioners and physician assistants receive.

After the initial medical evaluation, unaccompanied immigrant children are placed in holding areas, often with more than 100 children in each area; at this stage, they do not receive further medical attention unless they themselves alert CBP personnel, a nonmedical CBP staff member identifies a child in distress, or an adult caregiver reports an issue (in settings where they are allowed to stay with the child). Similarly, the *Juvenile Care Monitor Report* noted that when children have a contagious disease (e.g., COVID-19) requiring isolation, at some sites children were alone and in an area lacking appropriate staff supervision, and at others younger children were inappropriately housed with adolescents. Also, these isolation cells have been noted to become overcrowded, with only 1 advanced practice medical provider managing up to 125 children.[8]

Federal law requires screening to identify potential cases of trafficking. In an overzealous application of this mandate, when immigrant children are accompanied by a relative who is not a parent (e.g., adult sibling, cousin, or grandparent) and CBP apprehends them at the border, common practice is to separate the children from their family member, thus rendering them unaccompanied[13]; CBP may then deport the family member or send them to an adult immigrant detention facility.[8]

OFFICE OF REFUGEE RESETTLEMENT

Often within 72 hours, CBP transfers unaccompanied immigrant children to the custody of the ORR, where they are housed in 1 of more than 290 shelters across the country.[14] Within 48 hours of arrival to the shelter, they receive a physical examination, which is most often performed by a nurse practitioner or physician assistant (with the same limitations in extensive acute and chronic pediatric clinical training as noted); pediatricians may be onsite or available for consultation. Children receive limited medical, mental health, and maltreatment screenings, including for being trafficked. (A copy of the ORR medical and mental health screening form is on file with the authors and is available upon request.) Vaccinations are also initiated.[15]

Medical screening includes universal testing for tuberculosis and COVID-19 and urine pregnancy testing in postmenarchal females. Identified conditions requiring immediate medical care are addressed, which may involve transfer to a local hospital emergency department.[16] At the time of writing, unaccompanied immigrant children do not have the extensive medical and validated mental health screening evaluations recommended for newly arriving refugees, including children, per Centers for Disease Control and Prevention (CDC) refugee domestic screening guidance, even though they often have the same risk factors for infectious diseases, mental health concerns, and other diagnoses of significance.[14,17]

Children who arrive through formal US refugee resettlement pathways arrive legally, have formal medical screening initiated approximately 6 months before US arrival while in their refugee camp or in another site of displacement, and receive extensive medical and mental health screenings, most often within 30 days of US arrival.[17] Gaps in screening for unaccompanied immigrant children, compared with refugee children, include lack of testing for anemia, lead, eosinophilia, Strongyloides, other soil-transmitted helminth infections, vertical transmission of HIV, hepatitis B and C, and syphilis.

Unaccompanied immigrant children are only tested for sexually transmitted infections if they disclose sexual activity or abuse at arrival. Similarly, the children are only tested for blood-borne infections if they disclose injection drug use. Acute mental health interventions, treatments, referrals, and hospitalizations are only provided to unaccompanied immigrant children who have signs or disclose symptoms of severe depression, anxiety, or suicidal ideation. It is unlikely that detained children will disclose sensitive information, including sexual activity or abuse, intravenous drug use, trafficking, depression, anxiety, or suicidal ideation within 48 hours of arrival in an ORR shelter to clinicians who do not have a long-standing, trusting relationship; thus, underdiagnosing HIV, hepatitis B and C, syphilis, gonorrhea, and chlamydia and underidentifying children in need of more acute mental health services are likely.

If an unaccompanied immigrant child has a preexisting or newly diagnosed complex medical or mental health condition, before release from ORR custody ORR medical services staff ensure that linkage to a pediatrician and specialty follow-up care is established in or near the sponsor's community and arrange for medical or mental health records to be transferred to the accepting physician (per unpublished standards of ORR's Washington, DC, office and author experience). Thereafter, most children will be released to a parent or other "sponsor."[2] As of October 4, 2023, there were 10 818 unaccompanied immigrant children in HHS's care, and the average length of time an unaccompanied immigrant child remained in ORR's care was 24 days.[14]

RELEASE FROM FEDERAL CUSTODY

In calendar years 2021 and 2022, unaccompanied immigrant children were released to vetted sponsors, usually family members, with 11.8% and 14.0%, respectively, released to "distant relatives or nonfamily sponsors."[7,18] Sponsors are responsible for ensuring the child's ongoing safety and well-being and are advised to enroll the child in school, connect the child with a primary care medical home, and seek services from an immigration lawyer. Although sponsors are provided a copy of the child's ORR medical records at the time of discharge, the majority receive no federal or state oversight.[6,7] Unless the child is released in a state with Medicaid coverage for uninsured children—including those who are undocumented[19] or are identified as eligible for certain types of temporary legal status (e.g., victims of trafficking,[20] "special immigrant juveniles"[21])—they have limited access to health insurance once released from ORR custody.[19]

In fiscal year 2022, approximately 43% (55 900) of the nearly 130 000 unaccompanied immigrant children in ORR custody were deemed eligible for 4 months of postrelease services with a federally funded social worker to assist sponsors in linking the children to school, counseling, and legal, health, and mental health care.[14] There are no published criteria available that define which unaccompanied immigrant children are eligible for 4 months of social work support.

Also in fiscal year 2022, approximately 7% (9100) of the nearly 130 000 unaccompanied immigrant children in ORR custody had home studies to assess the home environment before release to a sponsor. However, recently updated ORR guidelines[14] require home studies for children identified as a victim of a severe form of trafficking (e.g., sex or labor trafficking), children with a diagnosed disability, children who have been identified as a victim of physical or sexual abuse "where the child's health or welfare has been significantly harmed or threatened," and children for whom there are concerns identified that the sponsor may pose a risk of abuse, maltreatment, exploitation, or trafficking.[14]

Home studies are also now newly required for any child who will be sent to live with a nonrelative sponsor who also will be hosting multiple children and when the child is aged 12 years or younger,[14] presumably in response to recent reports of unaccompanied immigrant children being labor trafficked by sponsors housing multiple unaccompanied immigrant children in nearly 50% of states.[6,7] These updated home study criteria require either that the traumatized child newly in the custody of CBP and ORR disclose they were sex or labor trafficked or physically or sexually abused or that a specific medical or mental health disability be diagnosed. These conditions may be easily missed if an extensively trained medical professional does not perform an appropriate medical-screening examination.

Released children are at high risk for trafficking and other abuse because of debt, familial poverty, lack of knowledge of US culture and labor laws, social isolation, marginalization, and other factors.[5] Based on their recent interviews of 60 caseworkers across the country, investigative journalists estimate that two thirds of unaccompanied immigrant children are working full-time and not in school; they found that the children were trafficked to work in meat plants, food packaging, contracting, and food delivery with no ongoing oversight of their health and well-being after release from ORR custody.[6,7]

Unaccompanied immigrant children and their sponsors face significant barriers to accessing ongoing health and mental health care.[22] Most children are released to states with no Medicaid coverage for undocumented immigrants,[19] and sponsors may not know where or how to receive discounted services.[22] Undocumented sponsors may avoid seeking care for fear of being identified and deported, and they may fear stigma associated with receipt of mental health services.[22] A national shortage of mental health providers further limits access for unaccompanied immigrant children and sponsors.[23] Most health care professionals have had no systematic training in evidence-based medical and trauma screening of immigrant populations,[24,25] including unaccompanied immigrant children, and are not aware of options to link unaccompanied immigrant children and their families to pro bono immigration assistance and resources for suspected trafficking. Barriers to legal services are exacerbated by a nationwide shortage of trained immigration lawyers who accept pro bono cases.[26]

Many of the existing legal protections unaccompanied immigrant children receive are the outcome of the 1997 *Flores Settlement Agreement* (*Flores*) and subsequent judicial enforcement orders in a 1985 class action lawsuit (*Flores v. Meese*). The Trump administration unsuccessfully sought to reduce DHS's obligations under *Flores* and sought to end the agreement. The Biden administration announced in December 2021 that it would not seek termination of the agreement.[8,27,28] Consistent with that approach, the Biden administration introduced proposed regulations in December 2023 that would largely codify the terms of *Flores* as they relate to ORR and HHS while explicitly noting that the settlement would remain in force for other federal agencies.[29]

The United States will continue to see arrivals of unaccompanied immigrant children, particularly from countries affected by instability, wars, famine, climate change, and poverty and those whose governments are unwilling or unable to adequately protect children. To address the needs of these children in a way that protects fundamental child rights, the US federal and state governments, along with input from experts in public health, law, and medicine, should take the following steps, among others.[30,31]

Federal funding should be allocated to do the following:

- Allow the development of systematic protocols for onboarding and frequent recertification of all medical providers staffing CBP and ORR facilities. This initiative should be led by pediatric physicians with expertise in immigrant health in the settings of primary care, emergency medicine, psychiatry, gynecology, behavior and development, child abuse, and infectious disease.
- Require CBP to have pediatric-trained medical providers deployed with them at all times to assist with immediate identification and medical triage of unaccompanied immigrant children at the border; they should also allow timely identification of acute and chronic medical issues.
- Allow daily around-the-clock on-call coverage by pediatric physicians (including pediatric psychiatrists) and trauma-trained pediatric psychologists to oversee and provide consultation for all pediatric-trained nurse practitioners, physician assistants, and masters-level counselors onsite at both CBP and ORR facilities, with provisions to address expected overcrowding. Pediatric physicians, psychiatrists, and psychologists should also provide weekly chart reviews.
- Require that all unaccompanied immigrant children have validated mental health screenings verbally administered at both CBP and ORR facilities and that children with positive screens be formally evaluated by a child psychologist or psychiatrist. Screens should be culturally adapted, suitable for unaccompanied immigrant children with limited literacy and available in Spanish and other commonly spoken languages.[32–34]
- Ensure that trauma-trained professional interpreters are available for children who do not speak English. As much as possible, bilingual medical providers should be recruited. Interpreters should be screened to ensure that they are not from a child's community and, where possible, are of a gender preferred by the child.
- Ensure that ORR medical screening includes all aspects of the CDC's refugee domestic screening guidance

used for refugee arrivals, including universal screening for HIV, hepatitis B, hepatitis C, syphilis, gonorrhea, chlamydia, Strongyloides, anemia, eosinophilia, and stool ova and parasites.[17]

- Support the design and implementation of a unified electronic medical record to facilitate appropriate interagency communication for all unaccompanied immigrant children similar to the interagency US Electronic Disease Notification system used for refugees accepted into the United States.[35]
- Expand the Unaccompanied Refugee Minor program to include all unaccompanied immigrant children who will not be released to a sponsor who is a known, trusted relative.[36] The Unaccompanied Refugee Minor program provides foster care, full CDC domestic refugee medical screening, ongoing site visits, assurance of school enrollment and attendance, and ongoing medical care.
- Ensure that all unaccompanied immigrant children are assigned a trained social worker for a minimum of 12 months of postrelease services who will link the child to full-time school, a medical home, mental health support, and local immigration nonprofits that support legal status applications. The service provider should work to ensure the child's safety and well-being, connecting them with local migrant and refugee organizations for support and facilitating successful integration into school.
- Address the national shortage of immigration lawyers by supporting the hiring of immigration lawyers by legal nonprofits to prioritize legal case representation of unaccompanied immigrant children.[37]
- Provide systematic training of community health care providers who serve immigrant children, particularly in federally qualified health centers[38,39] and systematic training of health care providers in pediatric emergency departments and hospitals, particularly at the border.
- Include information on the following:
    - CDC refugee domestic screening guidance[17];
    - trauma-informed, rights-based care[40];
    - specialized needs of immigrant children and families (e.g., health, mental health, legal, housing);
    - risk factors and potential indicators of child abuse and trafficking involving both labor and sex;
    - child abuse and trafficking screening strategies and appropriate responses, including reporting and referrals[5]; and
    - available community and national resources to address the specific needs of unaccompanied immigrant children and assist families as they adjust to their new conditions.
- Train, recruit, and retain mental health providers to systematically manage unaccompanied immigrant children during and after release.

In addition, the federal government should do the following:

- Provide the CDC Division of Global Migration Health with the authority to oversee all stages of health management of children arriving in the United States. Staff of this division write the CDC refugee domestic screening guidance[17] and are experts in the management of the health and welfare of refugee populations as well as the management of large surges of populations in crisis.
- Pass legislation that prohibits the separation of accompanied children from a trusted relative unless it is necessary for the safety of the child. This prevents children with families from being rendered unaccompanied.[30]
- Review the current sponsor vetting process and provide recommendations for improvement, with a specific focus on preventing child abuse, exploitation, and trafficking.
- Provide unaccompanied immigrant children with a card identifying them as unaccompanied, which should be presented to health professionals in any health setting. The card should include information for clinicians on how to obtain medical records from ORR[15] and summarize the special needs of this patient population.
- Ensure that all unaccompanied immigrant children being discharged from ORR care have a copy of all medical records and are verbally signed out by the ORR medical provider to a local federally qualified health center provider.[39] This involves ORR staff scheduling an appointment with a local federally qualified health center for an initial primary care visit before the child's discharge from ORR custody and ongoing oversite by the postrelease social worker.
- Ensure that sponsors and children of appropriate developmental age are provided standard written and recorded information in their preferred language. Topics should include the following:
    - state laws requiring children to attend school[41];

- laws regarding child labor and worker rights[42];
- labor and sex trafficking definitions, common recruitment strategies, and guidance on contacting the National Human Trafficking Resource Center for assistance (i.e., 1-888-373-7888; text: 233733)[43];
- how to apply for legal status and links to pro bono legal services[44];
- information to identify and link to federally qualified health centers with sliding scale programs for medical care[37]; and
- information for local medical providers on how to access children's medical records, including vaccine records,[15] and links to the CDC refugee domestic screening guidance[17] to ensure that patients receive all appropriate medical-screening evaluations and follow-up of abnormal results.

- Authorize courts to prioritize applications by unaccompanied immigrant children relating to their cases for special immigrant juvenile status, asylum, and other immigration status.

Implementing these changes is not without major challenges, particularly because immigration has become a polarizing political issue. Efforts will need to be made at public health, medical, and governmental levels to convey the value immigrants have for the US economy and society and the needs of unaccompanied immigrant children for ongoing public health support to foster successful integration; this will require strong national and state leadership, political and social will, and sufficient funding. Without these changes, unaccompanied immigrant children will remain at high risk for poor mental and physical health and dubious social outcomes, including being trafficked. Early and comprehensive attention to the needs of unaccompanied immigrant children maximizes the likelihood that they will reach their full potential and positively contribute to society. AJPH

ABOUT THE AUTHORS

Janine Young is with the University of California San Diego School of Medicine, Department of Pediatrics, La Jolla. Warren Binford is with the University of Colorado School of Medicine, Department of Pediatrics, Kempe Center, Center for Bioethics and Humanities, Aurora. Michael Garcia Bochenek is with Human Rights Watch, Children's Rights Division, New York, NY, and the Institute for the Study of Human Rights, Columbia University, New York, NY. Jordan Greenbaum is with the International Centre for Missing and Exploited Children, Alexandria, VA.

CORRESPONDENCE

Correspondence should be sent to Janine Young, MD, University of California San Diego School of Medicine, Department of Pediatrics, 7910 Frost St, 345, San Diego, CA 92123 (e-mail: jay028@health.ucsd.edu). Reprints can be ordered at http://www.ajph.org by clicking the "Reprints" link.

PUBLICATION INFORMATION

Full Citation: Young J, Binford W, Bochenek MG, Greenbaum J. Health risks of unaccompanied immigrant children in federal custody and in US communities. *Am J Public Health*. 2024;114(3):340–346.

Acceptance Date: December 21, 2023.

DOI: https://doi.org/10.2105/AJPH.2023.307570

CONTRIBUTORS

The author contributed equally to this essay.

ACKNOWLEDGMENTS

J. Young is supported by the Minnesota Center of Excellence in Newcomer Health (grant NU50CK000563 of the Centers for Disease Control and Prevention).

We dedicate this essay to our patients, clients, and their families.

CONFLICTS OF INTEREST

The authors have no conflicts of interest to declare.

REFERENCES

1. United Nations. Convention on the Rights of the Child. Available at: https://www.ohchr.org/en/instruments-mechanisms/instruments/convention-rights-child. Accessed October 26, 2023.
2. US Department of Health and Human Services. Unaccompanied children released to sponsors by state. September 28, 2023. Available at: https://www.acf.hhs.gov/orr/grant-funding/unaccompanied-children-released-sponsors-state. Accessed October 26, 2023.
3. United Nations. Children on the run—full report. Available at: https://www.unhcr.org/us/media/children-run-full-report. Accessed October 26, 2023.
4. Leyva-Flores R, Infante C, Gutierrez JP, Quintino-Perez F, Gómez-Saldivar M, Torres-Robles C. Migrants in transit through Mexico to the US: experiences with violence and related factors, 2009–2015. *PLoS One*. 2019;14(8):e0220775. https://doi.org/10.1371/journal.pone.0220775
5. Greenbaum J, Kaplan D, Young J, et al. Exploitation, labor and sex trafficking of children and adolescents: health care needs of patients. *Pediatrics*. 2023;151(1):e2022060416. https://doi.org/10.1542/peds.2022-060416
6. Dreier H, Luce K. Alone and exploited, migrant children work brutal jobs across the US. *New York Times*. February 25, 2023. Available at: https://www.nytimes.com/2023/02/25/us/unaccompanied-migrant-child-workers-exploitation.html. Accessed October 26, 2023.
7. Dreier H. As migrant children were put to work, US ignored warnings. *New York Times*. April 17, 2023. Available at: https://www.nytimes.com/2023/04/17/us/politics/migrant-child-labor-biden.html. Accessed October 26, 2023.
8. *Jenny Lisette Flores, et al., v. Merrick B. Garland*. Case no. CV 85-4544-DMG (2021). 2023. Available at: https://youthlaw.org/sites/default/files/2023-07/2023.01.30%20-%20Flores%20Juvenile%20Care%20Monitor%20Report.pdf. Accessed January 22, 2024.
9. Center For Human Rights & Constitutional Law. Mission statement. June 22, 2022. Available at: https://www.centerforhumanrights.org/who-we-are. Accessed January 22, 2024.
10. 8 CFR § 236.3 (2012). Available at: https://www.law.cornell.edu/cfr/text/8/236.3. Accessed October 26, 2023.
11. Liepert AE, Berndtson AE, Hill LL, et al. Association of 30-ft US–Mexico border wall in San Diego with increased migrant deaths, trauma center admissions, and injury severity. *JAMA Surg*. 2022;157(7):633–635. https://doi.org/10.1001/jamasurg.2022.1885
12. Velasco P. More than 14,000 asylum seekers were sent to San Diego. Local support systems were overwhelmed. *The Guardian*. October 19, 2023. Available at: https://www.theguardian.com/us-news/2023/oct/19/california-asylum-seekers-san-diego-budget-cuts. Accessed October 26, 2023.
13. Women's Refugee Commission. Protecting unaccompanied children: the Office of Refugee Resettlement (ORR) and the Trafficking Victims Protection Reauthorization Act (TVPRA). December 9, 2019. Available at: https://www.womensrefugeecommission.org/research-resources/protecting-unaccompanied-children-the-office-of-refugee-resettlement-orr-and-the-trafficking-victims-protection-reauthorization-act-tvpra. Accessed January 19, 2024.
14. US Department of Health and Human Services. Fact sheets and data. October 13, 2023. Available at: https://www.acf.hhs.gov/orr/about/ucs/facts-and-data. Accessed October 26, 2023.
15. US Department of Health and Human Services. ORR Unaccompanied Children Program policy

guide. Section 3. October 23, 2023. Available at: https://www.acf.hhs.gov/orr/policy-guidance/unaccompanied-children-program-policy-guide-section-3. Accessed October 26, 2023.

16. Administration for Children & Families. Medical services requiring heightened ORR involvement. September 29, 2020. Available at: https://www.acf.hhs.gov/sites/default/files/documents/orr/garza_policy_memorandum.pdf. Accessed October 31, 2023.
17. Centers for Disease Control and Prevention. Guidance for the US domestic medical examination for newly arriving refugees. March 30, 2023. Available at: https://www.cdc.gov/immigrantrefugeehealth/guidelines/domestic-guidelines.html. Accessed October 26, 2023.
18. US Department of Health and Human Services. More than 340 migrant kids sent to live with nonrelatives who sponsored other kids. June 2, 2023. Available at: https://www.nbcnews.com/politics/immigration/advocates-hhs-questions-unaccompanied-migrants-child-labor-rcna87326. Accessed October 26, 2023.
19. KFF. State-funded health coverage for immigrants as of July 2023. July 26, 2023. Available at: https://www.kff.org/racial-equity-and-health-policy/fact-sheet/state-funded-health-coverage-for-immigrants-as-of-july-2023. Accessed October 26, 2023.
20. US Citizenship and Immigration Services. Victims of human trafficking and other crimes. August 21, 2023. Available at: https://www.uscis.gov/humanitarian/victims-of-human-trafficking-and-other-crimes. Accessed October 26, 2023.
21. US Citizenship and Immigration Services. Special immigrant juveniles. March 31, 2023. Available at: https://www.uscis.gov/working-in-US/eb4/SIJ. Accessed October 26, 2023.
22. Hacker K, Anies M, Folb BL, Zallman L. Barriers to health care for undocumented immigrants: a literature review. *Risk Manag Healthc Policy*. 2015;8: 175–183. https://doi.org/10.2147/RMHP.S70173
23. Commonwealth Fund. Understanding the US behavioral health workforce shortage. May 8, 2024. Available at: https://www.commonwealthfund.org/publications/explainer/2023/may/understanding-us-behavioral-health-workforce-shortage. Accessed January 22, 2024. https://doi.org/10.26099/5km6-8193
24. Alpern JD, Davey CS, Song J. Perceived barriers to success for resident physicians interested in immigrant and refugee health. *BMC Med Educ*. 2016;16:178. https://doi.org/10.1186/s12909-016-0696-z
25. Bjorklund AB, Cook BA, Hendel-Paterson BR, Walker PF, Stauffer WM, Boulware DR. Impact of global health residency training on medical knowledge of immigrant health. *Am J Trop Med Hyg*. 2011;85(3):405–408. https://doi.org/10.4269/ajtmh.2011.10-0732
26. National Immigrant Justice Center. Access to counsel. Available at: https://immigrantjustice.org/issues/access-counsel. Accessed October 31, 2023.
27. Montoya-Galvez C. Biden administration discards Trump-era plan to end legal agreement protecting migrant children. December 11, 2021. Available at: https://www.cbsnews.com/news/biden-administration-discards-trump-era-plan-to-end-legal-agreement-protecting-migrant-children. Accessed January 19, 2024.
28. NPR. The history of the Flores Settlement and its effects on immigration. Available at: https://www.npr.org/2018/06/22/622678753/the-history-of-the-flores-settlement-and-its-effects-on-immigration. Accessed January 19, 2024.
29. US Department of Health and Human Services. Unaccompanied children program foundational rule. *Fed Regist*. 2023;88(191):68908–69002.
30. Linton JM, Griffin M, Shapiro AJ, et al. Detention of immigrant children. *Pediatrics*. 2017;139(5): e20170483. https://doi.org/10.1542/peds.2017-0483
31. Migration Policy Institute. Rising child migration to the United States. July 21, 2014. Available at: https://www.migrationpolicy.org/programs/us-immigration-policy-program/rising-child-migration-united-states. Accessed January 7, 2024.
32. Pathways to Wellness. Integrating refugee health and well-being. Available at: https://www.refugeehealthta.org/wp-content/uploads/2012/09/RHS15_Packet_PathwaysToWellness-1.pdf. Accessed October 26, 2023.
33. Minnesota Department of Health. WE-Check: Minnesota well-being and emotions check. December 30, 2021. Available at: https://www.health.state.mn.us/communities/rih/guide/wecheck.pdf. Accessed January 22, 2024.
34. Centers for Disease Control and Prevention. Guidance for mental health screening during the domestic medical examination for newly arrived refugees. August 30, 2022. Available at: https://www.cdc.gov/immigrantrefugeehealth/guidelines/domestic/mental-health-screening-guidelines.html. Accessed October 26, 2023.
35. Centers for Disease Control and Prevention. Electronic Disease Notification system. September 30, 2022. Available at: https://www.cdc.gov/immigrantrefugeehealth/Electronic-Disease-Notification-System.html. Accessed October 26, 2023.
36. US Department of Health and Human Services. Unaccompanied Refugee Minors Program. March 17, 2023. Available at: https://www.acf.hhs.gov/orr/programs/refugees/urm. Accessed October 26, 2023.
37. American Immigration Lawyers Association. Featured issue: ensuring legal representation for people facing removal. Available at: https://www.aila.org/advo-media/issues/featured-issue-ensuring-legal-representation. Accessed October 26, 2023.
38. Bureau of Primary Health Care. What is a health center? Available at: https://bphc.hrsa.gov/about-health-centers/what-health-center. Accessed October 26, 2023.
39. Health Resources and Services Administration. FQHCs and LALs by state. Available at: https://data.hrsa.gov/data/reports/datagrid?gridName=FQHCs. Accessed October 26, 2023.
40. Forkey H, Szilagyi M, Kelly ET, et al. Trauma-informed care. *Pediatrics*. 2021;148(2):e2021052580. https://doi.org/10.1542/peds.2021-052580
41. National Center for Education Statistics. State education practices. Available at: https://nces.ed.gov/programs/statereform/tab1_2-2020.asp. Accessed October 26, 2023.
42. US Department of Labor. State labor laws. Available at: http://www.dol.gov/agencies/whd/state. Accessed October 26, 2023.
43. National human trafficking hotline. Available at: https://humantraffickinghotline.org/en. Accessed October 26, 2023.
44. US Department of Justice. List of pro bono legal service providers. February 23, 2023. Available at: https://www.justice.gov/eoir/list-pro-bono-legal-service-providers. Accessed October 26, 2023.

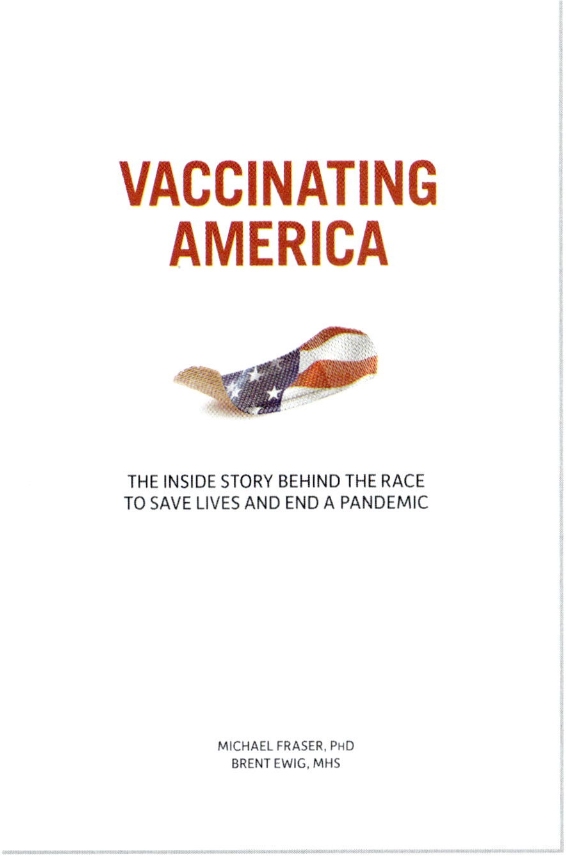

Vaccinating America: The Inside Story Behind the Race to Save Lives, and End a Pandemic

Edited by: Michael Fraser, PhD, Brent Ewig, MHS

2023, 250 PP, SFTCVR, ISBN 978-0-87553-332-2

Vaccinating America spotlights the public servants and heroes who planned and executed this unprecedented program to combat COVID-19 amidst fierce partisan divides, bureaucratic infighting and overwhelming logistical challenges, and doesn't hold back on pointing out those who hindered progress.

APHABOOKSTORE.ORG

APHA PRESS

AN IMPRINT OF AMERICAN PUBLIC HEALTH ASSOCIATION

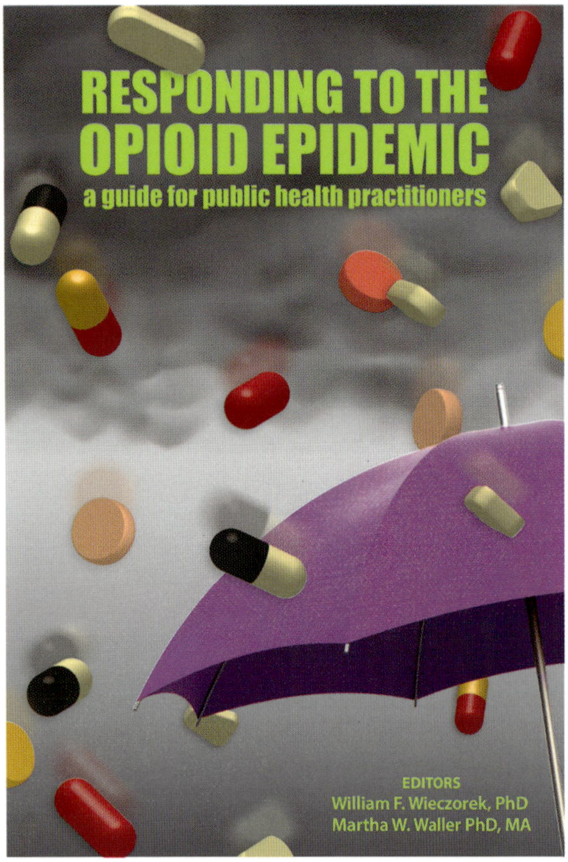

Responding to the Opioid Epidemic: A Guide for Public Health Practitioners

Edited by: William F. Wieczorek, PhD and Martha W. Waller PhD, MA

ISBN 978-0-87553-344-5, 400 PP., 2024,
SOFTBOUND/PRINT-ON-DEMAND

It's impossible to completely prevent the substance misuse defining the opioid epidemic, and it's impossible to treat the problem away. This reality requires a continuum of care (COC) approach, which includes promotion, prevention, case-finding, treatment, and recovery. This book presents research-informed interventions aligned with the COC approach to guide how communities, first responders, lay persons, medical providers, policymakers, treatment providers, and others can respond to the opioid epidemic at an individual, community, state, and national level.

APHABOOKSTORE.ORG

APHA PRESS

AN IMPRINT OF **AMERICAN PUBLIC HEALTH ASSOCIATION**